THE TRAUMA CHRONICLES

THE TRAUMA CHRONICLES

STEPHEN WESTABY

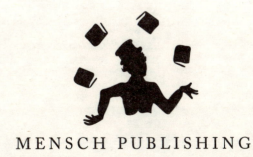

MENSCH PUBLISHING

Mensch Publishing
51 Northchurch Road, London N1 4EE, United Kingdom

First published in Great Britain 2023

Copyright © Stephen Westaby, 2023

Stephen Westaby has asserted his right under the Copyright, Designs and Patents Act, 1988, to be identified as Author of this work

All rights reserved. No part of this publication may be reproduced or transmitted in any form or by any means, electronic or mechanical, including photocopying, recording, or any information storage or retrieval system, without prior permission in writing from the publishers

A catalogue record for this book is available from the British Library

ISBN: HB: 978-1-912914-44-9; eBook: 978-1-912914-45-6

2 4 6 8 10 9 7 5 3 1

Typeset by Newgen KnowledgeWorks Pvt. Ltd., Chennai, India
Printed and bound in Great Britain by CPI Group (UK) Ltd, Croydon CR0 4YY

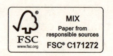

Dedications

Trauma ruthlessly destroys young lives. Accordingly, I dedicate this book to the paramedics, nurses, hospital doctors and surgeons who battle to save those with life-threatening injuries on a daily basis. More often than not it is our valiant police or fire service that initiates the process. It is stressful work that requires resilience.

Most of us support the principles of 'socialised medicine' but the NHS is not a sacred cow. It is there to be improved and that theme pervades my text. On occasions the opinions presented are controversial. Some may appear harsh, but criticism does not relate to valued individuals' rather to the circumstances that I continually sought to improve.

I owe a special tribute to a much admired Accident and Emergency nurse. Sister Sarah McDougall sympathetically tended to the rugby injuries of a bullish surgical trainee. Years later we married, after which Sarah saved me from myself. She is still the froth on the beer of my eventful career. Finally, nothing holds more importance for me than my children Gemma and Mark, and grandchildren Alice and Chloe. I constantly regret not spending more time with them, and suspect that most surgeons feel that way.

Some of the names of doctors, patients and the location of hospitals have been changed to preserve anonymity.

CONTENTS

Preface	ix
Introduction	1
Blood Bath	11
On the Road Again	27
Suspicious Minds	45
It Gets Difficult	65
Disappointment	89
Culture Shock	107
The American Way	131
Needless Deaths	149
'Scoop and Run' or 'Stay and Play'	171
Getting There	193
To Mend a Broken Heart	215
Right Place, Right Time	231
Trauma of a Different Kind	249
Postscript	273

PREFACE

A mind that is stretched by a new experience can
never go back to its old dimensions.

Oliver Wendell Holmes

As dismal though it might seem to others, I revelled in trauma surgery. I simply loved the unpredictability and urgency of it all. That race against time as life ebbs away. Me versus the Grim Reaper. That first incision into a crushed chest or swollen belly was like opening a Christmas present. But it was blood on my boots.

Consider the onslaught trauma provides for the senses. Shattered bones with deformed limbs. Horrific sights of guts and gore. Stressful sounds from the victim as life ebbs away then the pungent odour of antiseptics and spilled bodily fluids as we try to save them. What personal characteristics are needed to tackle major injuries on a daily basis? Where does the confidence come from to open someone's skull, thorax or abdomen when the appropriate specialists are not available. How does one dispense with normal human instincts in order to function impulsively? To operate without personal fear, inhibitions or empathy? Psychopaths do that.

In high pressure roles, epitomised by surgery and combat, the ability to make a decision in the midst of adversity goes with the territory. In his book *The*

PREFACE

Wisdom of Psychopaths the distinguished Oxford psychologist, Kevin Dutton, quotes a telling statement from a Navy Seal colonel. 'Should I think twice about pulling the trigger when the next thing to go through my head may well be from an AK-47?' The subtitle for Dutton's book reads: *What saints, spies and serial killers can teach us about success*, so I guess I came under the serial killers category. Despite my best efforts I lost scores of patients during a long career at the operating table. That said it was never without a fight. Desperate struggles to save the sick or salvage the mortally injured. I simply detested the misery and finality of death.

I first met Kevin Dutton when he chaired a packed house for me at the Cheltenham Literary Festival in the Autumn of 2019. The discussion went along the lines of *'what does it take to become a heart surgeon?* following as it did the publication of my book *The Knife's Edge.* An adviser for the special forces himself, Kevin had controversially ranked US President Donald Trump higher than Adolf Hitler on Hare's Psychopathy Diagnosis Checklist. This is how he introduced me in Cheltenham, then subsequently wrote in his next book *Black and White Thinking:*

> *Stephen Westaby is one of the world's great heart surgeons. And also one of the toughest. He headed up the Cardiothoracic Unit in Oxford for 30 years and took on operations that would have had other surgeons pissing their pants. Such was his dedication to the cause that Westaby pissed in his boots via a catheter, to maximise time at the table.' (That was a tale taken from my first book 'Fragile Lives').*
> *He garnered a reputation in less staid bureaucratic*

PREFACE

*times as a swashbuckling braggadocio, wielding
scalpel and saw in his rugby kit, blasting out Pink
Floyd. A diagnosed psychopath, he cruised darkened
hospital corridors in the wee small hours like
some kind of ruthless, predatory anti-serial killer,
stalking the Grim Reaper to within an inch of his
life, spoiling for fights and cooking up reasons and
pretexts as he went. If he was fortunate enough to
find any he usually emerged victorious.*

'Thanks for that, Kevin,' I murmured under my breath. Needless to say, that graphic introduction sensitised the delicate gentlefolk in the Cheltenham audience to what was coming next. I began reasonably enough, explaining that those who distinguish themselves in surgery must be decisive and stand out in the heat of the battle. But then I illustrated the point with pictures of a gory chest transfixion case which prompted a crash and a commotion in the midst of what had, until then, been a hushed audience. A sensitive soul had fainted, toppling noisily from his chair and lay crumpled in a heap on the floor.

Afterwards, in the Green Room, I told my new psychologist friend about the textbooks I had published on major trauma and he suggested that I should write some of the tales for the general public. 'A lot of people would want to read a book like that,' he said. 'There are more psychos around than you realise. My special forces mates would love it.'

Curiously enough, I credited my particular surgical persona to a head injury of my own. It was the sexist swinging 60s when I was just nineteen. The concept of being 'woke' didn't exist in those days. As a shy backstreet kid from Scunthorpe who had worked at the steelworks, it was apparent that if I was going to get on at a London medical school I had to play rugby. It happened that I had a flair for the game but, on a cold winter's afternoon on tour in Cornwall, an opponent's boot rendered me instantly unconscious. I was left lying face down in a muddy puddle while my illustrious team mates frantically pursued the ball down the pitch. What was more important to them, beating the local yokels or resurrecting their colleague? The former of course, but a blow to the head followed by oxygen deprivation is a particularly dangerous combination.

Nursing a battered, swollen brain I was transferred from the local hospital in Truro to the old Charing Cross Hospital on Strand. There it became apparent that the modest retiring young student had personality changes. So much so that the hospital discharge letter reported that I had been 'aggressive towards doctors, promiscuous with the night nurses and generally lacking of inhibitions and demeanour.' According to Kevin, I manifest the Phineas Gage phenomenon from the classic textbooks of psychology. In the rail engineer's case, exploding dynamite had driven a tamping iron through his skull and frontal lobes. Disinhibited and outrageous, he was eventually admitted to a lunatic asylum. As for myself, within weeks I was elected medical school social secretary and compere for the Christmas shows. Liberated from shyness and self-doubt, I graduated with the award of 'student most likely to succeed'.

Disinhibition and boldness were welcome characteristics for a surgical career but in other respects my Phineas phenomenon proved catastrophic. Relationships suffered. Having qualified as a doctor,

PREFACE

I married my childhood sweetheart from the grammar school. By then, Jane was a vivacious Cambridge-trained teacher whose last interest in the world was guts and gore. And sadly for both of us, the introverted medical student from Scunthorpe morphed into a flamboyant testosterone-fuelled 'wannabe' surgeon who spent alternative nights and weekends resident in the hospital. Sadly lacking in principles at that stage, this perpetual insomniac would do just what Dutton suggested—stalk corridors at night but in the nurses' home, seeking out parties and any port in an androgen storm. Jane didn't deserve that.

Infidelity seemed to be a knife wielder's personality trait back in those days since several of my colleagues' marriages ended abruptly for the same reasons. None of us were proud of the fact—very much the opposite—but at least I had the brain trauma to blame. In contrast the trainee physicians, in general, had a palpably different mindset. With fewer rugby players they were predominantly intellectuals with more self-esteem and less bravado. It had always been that way. In the eighteenth century the College of Physicians would not countenance membership for the uncouth 'Barber surgeons.' The gaggle of misfits who chopped off legs without anaesthetic had to launch their own establishment in Lincoln's Inn Fields little more than a mile away in the City. At least they were close to the lawyers there to keep them out of trouble.

I vividly recall failing the Fellowship of the Royal College of Surgeons on the first attempt. The names of the few successful candidates were called out loudly in the entrance hall next to the statue of John Hunter the anatomist. The newly accredited surgeons were invited

PREFACE

to enter the hallowed halls to collect their swanky certificates. The chaff, or body snatchers as I called us, wandered off into Fleet Street for a few dreary pints in consolation.

Fast forward ten years to 1978. Fulfilling the promise of my optimistic award I was now a budding young surgical trainee with the famous transplant surgeon Sir Roy Calne in Cambridge. Calne was a competitive tennis player who enjoyed having sporty trainees on his team. He encouraged me to carry on playing rugby, which I did, causing frequent visits to the Addenbrookes Hospital Accident Department. One grim winter's afternoon found me sitting sorrowfully in sisters' office wearing muddy kit and waiting for an orthodontic surgeon to scrutinise my skull X-rays. Just before Christmas, I had sustained an unpleasant jaw fracture that sheared off the roots of a molar tooth and was garnering sympathy from the student nurses. Then in rushed the boss, Sister Sarah McDougall, who urged me to follow her to the Emergency room. Given that I would happily follow this beautiful woman to the ends of the earth, I found myself at the centre of one of the most taxing situations of my career to date.

A young man had been injured in a high speed motor cycle crash rendering him unconscious with bleeding into his left chest. The duty anaesthetist had attached him to a ventilator and was pouring in fluids, yet the blood pressure kept falling. There were no chest surgeons at Addenbrookes but sister knew that I had worked in heart surgery at the Brompton Hospital. Would I try to help, irrespective of the muddy knees? So I did.

Pulling on a surgical gown over the rugby kit, I proceeded to slice him open between the ribs while

PREFACE

spitting my own blood into the scrub sink behind me. Unfortunately, he had transected his aorta, the largest blood vessel in the body and grasping it with my fist just wasn't enough. He died in a torrent of bleeding which gushed all over me, but at least I had tried my best under the circumstances. When the orthodontic surgeon arrived in the midst of this he was told 'Westaby is in the Emergency room with a chest open.' Visibly shocked, the man thought he had arrived too late, that I had inhaled the broken tooth and it was me they were trying to resuscitate.

That fractured jaw did serve one useful purpose. It stopped me talking my way out of a pass mark for the final Fellowship of the Royal College of Surgeons viva, as I had done on the previous occasion. After huge operative experience in the abdomen, I switched to training as a heart surgeon. Yet not a single minute in Cambridge was wasted, whether operating on guts, gall bladders or genitals. Delicate manipulation of the instruments, gentle handling of the tissues and sound surgical judgement only come with experience. Hour after hour of cutting and stitching. Surgery is an apprenticeship just like carpentry or decorating. And to operate on a moving target requires skill. Believe me, the manual dexterity and confidence to operate on a child's heart cannot be gained through books, podcasts or computer simulation despite what contemporary leaders might tell you. Time at the coal face is what counts.

An affinity for trauma surgery never did divert my focus from the heart. But throughout my career I enthusiastically strove to rescue the injured, particularly when Oxford emerged as one of the country's first major trauma centres. What's more, through visiting

xv

PREFACE

trauma units in the US, South Africa and Asia I learned many useful surgical techniques. I vividly recall being in a Tokyo accident department and watching a trauma surgeon slice open the left chest to clamp the aorta above the diaphragm. His colleagues were attempting to stop torrential bleeding from a pulped liver in a construction worker who had fallen from a tall building. The simple manoeuvre cut off the blood supply to the lower half of the body and instantly turned off the tap. Sadly, there was not enough liver left and he died despite the heroics; but I used the method later, successfully, to benefit injured patients in Oxford.

After the success of *Fragile Lives* and *The Knife's Edge* I needed encouragement to write a third biography. Yet with a leading psychologist expressing enthusiasm about the story lines what else should I do during the Covid lockdown? The theme is about making things better. When my medical career began in the 1970s, the severely injured were simply conveyed by ambulance to the nearest district general hospital with a casualty department. There was no pre-hospital care and the patients were generally received by recently qualified doctors who were ill-equipped to manage multiple injuries. There were trainee abdominal and orthopaedic surgeons on call but, more often than not, they were sequestered away with their bosses in an operating theatre or outpatients clinic. Meanwhile, the victim continued to bleed to death. Worse still, the specialist brain and chest surgeons were located in separate hospitals that could only be accessed secondarily. That was, however, useful from my standpoint. As a disinhibited and aggressive young surgeon I had a free hand to zip open any part

PREFACE

of the body in an attempt to save a life. And that's what I did. I simply hated to lose a patient then try to explain that to a grieving family. Nevertheless, it was clear to me that this appalling situation must change and I consider myself privileged by being able to play a small part in making that happen. This is an account of that journey.

To save a life is a wonderful thing but, as I will eventually explain, the macho swashbuckling surgical stereotype of the twentieth century no longer exists, so my stories relate to a bygone era. In these times of equality and diversity, surgeons have defined working hours like any other profession. Their training is shorter and they micro specialise in one part of the body. Don't expect a gut surgeon to open a chest, or a heart surgeon to drill into the skull. Don't anticipate that a kidney surgeon is qualified to operate on the stomach. Those days have gone and perhaps that's a good thing. So make sure you find the right specialist when you need one and, when you get into a car, please don't forget to fasten your seat belt.

xvii

Introduction

Life is not fair – get used to it!

Bill Gates

Spring 1980, at Harefield Hospital on a Saturday morning. I was perched on a stool in an operating theatre, triumphantly extracting a peanut from an infant's bronchial tubes. I had deftly manoeuvred the rigid brass bronchoscope through the child's voice box so the narrow, dimly lit aperture of the instrument was situated deeply within his tiny chest. Not dissimilar to sword swallowing. Just as I located the foreign body, theatre sister poked her head through the anaesthetic room door. Sensing her presence, I made every effort not to divert from purpose as the grasping forceps slipped down through the dark tunnel. But Sister's perfume was more powerful than the anaesthetic gases.

Ever persistent, she coughed intentionally then tapped on the door through which she had already entered. 'Sorry to interrupt Steve, but the switchboard have just called. They say you're needed in theatre at Wycombe as soon as you can get there. Apparently the doctor said not to waste time calling back. Just get there as quickly as you can.' With those last few words my concentration evaporated. I squeezed the peanut too hard in the jaws of the forceps and it disintegrated. Oily fragments vanished into small airways beyond reach. While the phrase 'oh shit' reverberated through my cerebral cortex, what I uttered in a controlled manner was 'what I can't hoover out through the sucker the kid will just have to cough up. It sounds as if I need to go.'

At thirty-two, I was a restless, ruthlessly ambitious adrenaline junkie, hyper-focused on becoming a heart surgeon. Marriage number one was in tatters through my own misdemeanours and I had arrived at Harefield with a suitcase packed with clothes and books. Nothing else. No home, no car. I lived on the job in hospital accommodation and was always available. I actually needed to be. The specialist hospital covered an enormous area of North London and the home counties for chest surgery emergencies. From the Central Middlesex and Northwick Park hospitals on the periphery of the city to the towns of High Wycombe, Hemel Hempstead and St Albans to the North. From Slough and Windsor in the west to Watford and Barnet in the east. Many acute hospitals with an accident department were served by Harefield. Some of them held a thoracic surgery outpatients clinic once or twice a month so, as an itinerant practitioner, I did at least know where to find them. That said I had never worked outside a posh teaching hospital so the reality of operating on emergencies at St Elsewhere's came as a culture shock.

In those days, specialist surgeons had to complete general surgery training first which I had done happily in Cambridge. Not uneventfully, I might add, but I did eventually pass the exams. Budding cardiac surgeons then had to spend time operating on the lungs and gullet, predominantly for cancer. For me, these structures were far less compelling than the beautiful

INTRODUCTION

heart in continuous motion, a magical organ to watch and repair. Spongy lungs just inflated and deflated like my prolific private parts, but a little more often, I guess. Yet with a knife or needle holder in my hand, I was happy. I was a compulsive operator who sought solace in the operating theatre away from my complicated personal life. Enough said. But surgical training seemed to go on forever and the tedium of extracting peanuts from bronchial tubes at weekends was as compelling as a poke in the eye with a sharp stick.

My immediate bosses at Harefield were two distinguished, if not eccentric, chest surgeons who were cruising towards retirement. The senior thoracic surgeon, John Jackson, was a kindly Irishman, the son of a Canon of St Patrick's Cathedral in Dublin. When his wayward apprentice arrived by bus carrying all his belongings, he was quick to insist that I needed wheels. So he drove me to see one of his grateful cancer patients, a motor dealer in North London. I left with a beat up blue MG at surprisingly little cost, which I guess was a charitable contribution towards the humanitarian mission that I was expected to follow.

The second was Mary Shepherd, one of the singularly rare breed of female cardiothoracic surgeons in those days. A distinctive if not curious character, she was a spinster, drove a white Jaguar saloon and smoked like a chimney. In the Lung Cancer Clinic she would sit coughing and grinning like a Cheshire cat while I pointedly preached to the patients about giving up the filthy habit. Mary cheerfully let me do all the work while she served on the board of Wormwood Scrubs prison. She often alluded to the fact that I belonged in that institution, rather than in the power base of my training rotation, the famous Hammersmith Hospital next door.

I got on well with both of them and, as such, their solitary senior registrar was willingly granted free rein for all trauma calls throughout this huge region. It was a privileged situation in an era when major injuries were more of an inconvenience than a priority for the NHS. In those days, there were no coordinated systems in place for trauma care. Orthopaedic surgeons fixed broken bones and general surgeons explored abdominal injuries all in their own general hospitals. Sometimes bleeding brains reached a neurosurgery unit but often they didn't. It was the same for chest injuries. But Harefield had just started a heart transplant programme and the immunosuppressed recipients were kept isolated amidst routine surgery patients in the small intensive care unit. Admission of chest trauma patients from other hospitals was simply not an option. So I dealt with them where I found them.

Harefield Hospital is in a curious location for a regional cardiothoracic unit, particularly one that aspired to become the world's most prolific heart transplant centre. Down a narrow winding country lane in north Middlesex lies an undistinguished village and what used to be the magnificent Harefield Park Estate overlooking the Colne Valley and Grand Union Canal. At the turn of the twentieth century, the land was owned by a wealthy Australian sheep farmer called Charles Billyard-Leake who lived in a fine seventeenth century manor house surrounded by lake, stables and coach house. Decades later, I was living in his palatial bedroom on the mansion's third floor overlooking the construction of the M25 motorway.

At the outbreak of World War I, the philanthropic Leake offered his grand country house to the Australian Government as a refuge for wounded soldiers evacuated from France and Belgium. The property was soon oversubscribed and surrounded by temporary wooden huts and canvas tents appropriately renamed the Number 1 Australian Auxiliary Hospital. It eventually housed two thousand war casualties far from home. When the War ended, the buildings were taken over by Middlesex County Council who turned them into a tuberculosis hospital. At the dizzy heights of 290 feet above sea level, the facility supposedly offered fresh air and sunlight favoured for the recovery of infected lungs. New three storey brick buildings were then built with flat roofs, glass-sided corridors and balconies for the patients to sit outside in the sunshine. The ground plan resembled a seagull with its wings spread wide. The main entrance was, and still is, at the beak with a concert hall opposite. Operating theatres were built at the rear when chest surgery was developed to treat the onerous complications of tuberculosis.

During World War II, Harefield was used as a casualty station for victims of the Blitz alongside St Mary's Hospital in Paddington. As such, the facilities were converted into a general hospital which was taken over by the NHS at its inception in 1948. It was then that cardiac surgery developed as a specialty, following the audacious removal of shrapnel and bullets from the heart's chambers at the US Military Field Hospital in the Cotswolds. Progress in lung surgery at Harefield ultimately led to pioneering procedures on the heart by Sir Thomas Holmes Sellors.

There were distinct similarities between Harefield and Papworth Hospital where I had started my surgical training in Cambridge. During World War II the Papworth Village Settlement was also a countryside sanatorium for solders with tuberculosis. Fifteen miles from Addenbrookes Hospital in the city, it also evolved into a centre for chest medicine, then cardiology, then cardiothoracic surgery and ultimately cardiac transplantation. It was after Papworth that I became Professor Sir Roy Calne's registrar in Cambridge. That was soon after he began a pioneering liver transplant programme alongside kidney transplantation at Addenbrookes which was supported by the University's research on the immunosuppressive drug cyclosporin.

I recall the heated discussions in Cambridge about restarting heart transplants in the UK after Donald Ross was stopped from doing them in London. Despite the fact that cardiac surgery was based out at Papworth, Calne wanted all transplantation to be done within an established service. What was more important, he argued, the straightforward plumbing that took a couple of hours, or the ongoing complexity of organ rejection that claimed so many lives and brought a halt to the original attempts? But it was not to be.

Britain's cardiac transplants, which began at the National Heart Hospital in London, were resumed at two isolated tuberculosis sanatoria in the countryside. It was a personality thing, not strategic planning. There was no NHS strategy. The surgeons simply declared 'we're going to transplant hearts here' and so they did. I did precisely the same when I came to develop mechanical hearts as an alternative in Oxford—blood pumps that can be taken from the shelf, and operations that are not reliant upon a supply of head injury patients.

INTRODUCTION

Did I relish being out in the sticks operating on lung and oesophageal cancer? To be honest, no. There were no CT or MRI scans in 1980. Just plain chest X-rays. So if there was no obvious spread on the black and white image we would proceed to remove what was obvious. Frequently there was much cancerous growth that was not visible and the poor patient was doomed from the outset. Large, painful incision between the ribs, no benefit. Thankfully, everything is different now, but at the time it was depressing. And I was a restless soul, easily bored. So after months of carving out cancer I took myself off to Hong Kong Island as a locum consultant in general surgery to test what I had learned in Cambridge. Then a public hospital in Kowloon asked whether I would do some chest surgery for them on a charitable basis. More than delighted to do so, I was exposed to a variety of fascinating problems that I would never deal with in the West.

Besides supreme confidence, I brought another contribution back to Harefield which proved immediately controversial. Professor Guan Bee Ong at the Hong Kong University Hospital taught me the seemingly outrageous but relatively safe technique of stripping out the whole gullet using finger dissection and without opening the chest. No painful cuts between the ribs, just a short incision in the neck and a second in the upper abdomen to mobilise the stomach. I then made the stomach into a tube, to be joined up to a stump of residual oesophagus in the neck. Magic. One of my bosses, Mr Jackson, arranged for me to demonstrate this less invasive procedure to a gathering of thoracic surgeons in London, but predictably none adopted the intimidating technique. Most were too worried to try it and I was quietly deemed a reckless young man. And so I was. There was a reason that would only reveal itself much later in life.

Genuinely concerned for my future, kindly Mr Jackson invited me to his home for a quiet word. 'Westaby,' he said 'there's something different about you and I'm trying to work out what it is. There are hoops to jump through in this business and those who make it have to fit in. You're a natural operator. You perform way above your station in that respect but you antagonise people. They won't want you as a colleague, then you won't get the jobs you deserve.'

At that point I told him about the head injury during medical school. That fateful blow to the head on the rugby pitch that changed my personality. The abrupt change from self-consciousness and introspection to lack of inhibitions and fearlessness. Surely that was the basis for a successful surgical career once I could stop bowing and scraping to my bosses? But I didn't vocalise that last bit. I just smiled and chirped 'It's really not my fault I'm different. Blame the Cornish farmer who kicked me in the head!' Jackson smiled and I suspect he finally reached the point of the whole discussion. 'You would of course be welcome here. Both Mary and I are going to retire in a couple of years. That should be just when you finish your training.'

'That's very kind of you to suggest it,' is what I said, but I had no intention of staying in thoracic surgery. I needed to get back to hearts. Nonetheless the warm endorsement settled me down a bit after my escapades in the Far East.

Though I preferred to be at the Hammersmith or Great Ormond Street, Harefield had a charm of its own.

INTRODUCTION

I had the manor house with a bar to live in, then two supportive bosses who, having seen it all and done it all, were only too pleased to let me operate on their cases. The staff were largely local folk and friendly, as they tend to be in smaller hospitals. There were cosy country pubs close by with log fires and country bumpkins to impress with tales of blood and gore. When called across to the wards at night, I would invariably encounter a fox, a badger or a deer roaming the grounds, and the owls would screech at me. And at that stage of my career, I had free rein over the trauma surgery. No one else wanted to do it.

Blood Bath

Believe in yourself. You are braver than you think,
more talented than you know, and capable of more
than you imagine.

Roy T. Bennett

The Theatre Sister had conveyed the air of desperation from Wycombe rather well. I got the message. So much so that I didn't change out of blues or take my jacket. Blue scrubs to blue car and off I went. With precariously fine, if not reckless, judgement there was just enough petrol in the tank to carry me the 15 miles, and on a weekend in the sunshine it felt good to be out on the road.

Saturday morning shoppers meandered across the main street of this sleepy hollow as I turned right from the hospital gates. Unlike police cars or ambulances, I had no blue light or siren on the MG. No way of explaining that grave sense of urgency. Given the note of despair in the call, the patient's projected survival was short. Had they not needed emergency surgery they wouldn't have called us. So I drove with the disregard for other road users that had been routine in Hong Kong. Blasting the squeaky horn so everyone considered me a complete idiot. Once free from the village I let rip with a sense of freedom, pushing the spent sports car as fast as I could go towards the Oxford Road.

There were several police cars around the entrance to the accident department offering clues to what lay ahead. In the hushed reception area, I asked for directions to the operating theatres. The nurse asked me 'are you the chest surgeon from Harefield?' When I responded in the affirmative, she replied 'take the lift to the second floor and the theatres are signposted. Hope you're in time. Best of luck with the poor woman.'

The curtains were ajar in one of the emergency bays which was empty. No trolley, but lots of discarded swabs and pools of dried blood on the floor. More drops of blood marked a trail to the lifts, one of which was marked 'out of order.' I surmised that it was being cleaned, questioning whether my mercy dash was already futile. At that point I was overtaken by a porter carrying bags of blood who decided to run up the stairs. I followed. On the second floor, a uniformed policeman stood silently at the entrance to the operating theatre corridor. Waving me through, the officer blandly offered 'they're in theatre 2, Sir,' so perhaps the patient was still alive.

The automatic doors swung open as if by telepathy and there, under the operating lights, was the anaesthetist frantically squeezing cold blood straight from the fridge into a drip. I knew that because the energetic porter had just handed the plastic bag to her. Cold is not great in such circumstances but needs must. By now I had reached the conclusion that this must be something pretty unpleasant but when the crowds parted for 'the hero from Harefield' even I was caught off guard. Blood-soaked underwear discarded in haste now littered the floor beneath the table. It had been cut away from her young body to expose the many wounds. My gaze was drawn to the letter 'T' carved deeply and deliberately into her abdominal wall, the gaping subcutaneous fat shining golden yellow under the bright lights. Then there were multiple stab wounds in the front of her neck and chest. At least two were situated directly over the heart. This was obviously meant to be a ritualistic murder attempt, but Harefield took the call an hour before and I wondered why she wasn't already dead.

In a room pervaded by doom and gloom the computer between my ears was trying to process stuff. Blood pressure 70/50 thereabouts, and heart rate 136. I wanted to know the pressure in her veins but they didn't have a line in for that. She was deathly pale despite the blood transfusion and both cold and sweaty to touch. This was bog standard haemorrhagic shock but with a cardiac twist. I was sure the knife had penetrated at least the right side of the heart but blood must have accumulated and clotted within its fibrous bag, the pericardial sac, thus curtailing the bleeding. We call that cardiac tamponade and it's critically important not to overfill the circulation and blow those clots out of the stab wounds. I knew that, but non-cardiac folk often don't. They just keep on trying to restore a respectable blood pressure which is not possible under the circumstances.

Something else was really troubling me. The anaesthetist hadn't tried to insert a tracheal tube to secure her airway. What's more I could hear gas hissing out of the girl's neck from the wound in her throat. That meant that the knife had severed the windpipe, but to what degree? My anaesthetist ally in this struggle didn't want to risk pushing her plastic tracheal tube past the wound in case the lacerated ends of the pipe separated. Then the ability to ventilate would be lost altogether.

So she was blowing in oxygen and anaesthetic gases through a black rubber face mask. Some of it must have been reaching the victim's lungs but we were breathing the rest. My computer told me one more thing. The belly was distended. Either it was also full of blood, which I suspected, or she was in an advanced state of pregnancy which the Wycombe folk surely must have considered already. If that was the case it would be imperative to deliver the baby quickly. Placenta's don't cope well in shock.

While working that lot out I was not saying very much and was trying hard not to be critical. I just said 'don't give her any more cold blood or clear fluid right now. It just buggers up the clotting. Let me open her up and get control of the bleeding. But first things first. Do you have a bronchoscope? And a set of oesophageal bougies?' I needed to get that tracheal tube down through her injured windpipe so at least the airway and breathing was under control. 'And have you done a chest X-ray?' The two questions generated frenzied but purposeful activity from the anxious nurses. Where was the bronchoscope kept? No one ever used it. Then the chest X-ray had been left down in the accident department, which was no bloody good to me. I dispatched the house officer from the duty surgical firm at top speed to retrieve it.

Where was the consultant general surgeon on call? Had anyone senior taken an interest in this potential homicide? The call had been taken on the golf course. The response 'you need a cardiothoracic surgeon, not me. Call Harefield.' Life was like that in the old days. The locum anaesthetist, Wendy Wu, was left to do her best on the resuscitation front and wisely decided to bring the poor victim directly to the operating theatre hoping that a surgeon would follow. It was the right call in the circumstances. But no more transfusion now. The time for more blood was when I had stopped it pissing out of the heart and major blood vessels.

The bronchoscope was ready and, mercifully, its light source worked when the theatre orderly eventually remembered to plug it in. Clearly it was the first time out of its box for many years. Wendy was wobbly about what to expect so I politely instructed her to hyperventilate the leaky lungs for a while using the face mask, then let me take over. Ignoring the gaping wounds I tipped the young woman's head back, pushed her chin forward and slid the rigid scope over the tongue to the back of her throat. Blood and secretions filled the end of the copper tube as it grated against her teeth, then everything went dark.

After sucking vigorously on blood and mucus I recognised the cartilaginous epiglottis guarding the entrance to the voice box. The vocal chords twitched nervously as I approached and, in a second, I was through them. The dark, D-shaped tube ahead was the windpipe clogged with old blood and as I sucked all that away, there, about a third of the way down, was the knife wound. A cut of around 50% of the circumference. On appearance, I judged it unlikely to disrupt if I passed through the flexible bougie then railroaded the stiff tracheal tube over it. That was an easy manoeuvre compared with fishing for peanuts in a small child's bronchial tree. Once deep into the windpipe I asked Wendy to blow up the balloon surrounding the distal part of the tube. That ensured that gas went south into the lungs rather than leaking backwards around it. Then she could secure the whole thing so it couldn't displace from the airway during surgery.

When I turned to Wendy, she was visibly trembling. And who could blame her. She had a good idea what I was about to do next and was mightily apprehensive. It was no more reassuring when I enquired if they had internal defibrillating paddles. So I quizzed her directly, 'have you ever done any cardiac surgery?' She let her mask drop for the first time to open a stubborn bottle top with her teeth. 'No' she murmured. Pumped up with adrenaline and testosterone as I was by now, I thought she was very attractive. Did that make a difference? It shouldn't, but it did.

The rigid NHS hierarchy was reversed here. The trainee needed to take charge and she knew it. Yet as my only help in an attempt to prevent a murder we needed a calm and mutually supportive working relationship for the next few hours. Then if we saved the victim perhaps we would drive off into the sunset, to Henley or Marlow, for a drink. Even in these appalling circumstances it was Saturday evening and I could easily be distracted by a beautiful woman. It was the old days of overt sexism in surgery, I'd be expelled instantly these days like a naughty schoolboy.

I painted the body with iodine from chin to pubic bone, driving the sponge deeply into the many contaminated wounds in an attempt to clean them. While clipping the green drapes to her skin the houseman returned with the chest X-ray and displayed it on the light box on the wall. Most of the story was revealed by that one picture. A globular-shaped heart shadow took my attention first. To the tutored eye, there was a substantial collection of blood clot around the heart and this explained the low blood pressure despite many litres of transfused fluid. Then there was blood and air in the right side of the chest consistent with a second, deeply penetrating wound. I felt that the partially obscured diaphragm on the left side was pushed upwards by blood in the abdomen, then as expected there was free air in the subcutaneous tissues of the neck.

Wendy Wu asked me what I planned to do given the appearances. I told her I intended to open the poor girl from neck to umbilicus straight down the midline. I would repair the heart first then work my way through the other wounds depending upon what was bleeding fastest. We also had to repair the leaking windpipe but that was under control and could wait until last. Now I sensed that the poor perspiring scrub nurse was way out of her depth.

I couldn't see a sternal saw in their tray of surgical instruments. In cardiac centres, we run an oscillating saw up the length of the breast bone then spread the edges wide with a metal retractor. The theatre sister had laid out just about every retractor known to man for me to choose from but I could see no saw. 'Sorry but we don't have one, I could only find the old fashioned chisel and mallet. We don't do any heart surgery here.' Of course she didn't have to tell me that. The reality was that I must operate on neck, chest and abdomen, in a potential murder case, in an unfamiliar environment, with a disparate group whom I had never previously encountered. No problem. I had done it in Hong Kong, I would manage in High Wycombe.

I had never bisected a breast bone with hammer and chisel before, but that was OK. At least there was something to use. Wendy pointed out that the blood pressure had started to drift down again, having stopped the transfusion. So I took the scalpel from my helper's shaking hand and ran it through skin and fat for a good eighteen inches. There was little bleeding given the girl's deeply shocked state — her superficial blood vessels had constricted to divert blood to the vital organs. This anticipated finding prompted me to ask Wendy Wu, 'Is she acidotic?' The level of acid in the circulation is an index of whether the muscles and internal organs are receiving sufficient blood flow. It was Wendy's own assistant, the anaesthetic nurse, who responded. 'Yes, very.' The last pH was 6.9.

'Shit' I responded. 'Do you think we should give her some bicarbonate.'

'Already done it' said Wendy. 'I'm repeating the blood gases and haemoglobin level now.'

My blade went much deeper on second pass. Directly down onto the breast bone and abdominal muscles but still no oozing. Moving on at pace I rammed my index finger up under the bone to give access to my primitive instrument. The stainless steel chisel, a museum piece, had a sharp advancing blade and a blunt guard at the lower end to protect the tissues beneath. The objective was to keep it aligned with the midline of the sternum while a metal mallet bashed it along, spattering bone marrow in its wake. A saw takes five seconds, the chisel fifty-five. Most of that time was spent assiduously maintaining its alignment towards the neck.

With bisected bone spread widely the story unfolded amidst mounting excitement. The glistening pericardial sac was indeed distended. It had that dark purple cardiac tamponade appearance with blood clot like liver protruding from the tell-tale knife wound. Despite intense focus I couldn't fail to be aware of noisy happenings behind me. While Wendy's gaze remained firmly fixed on the pathology in front of us, the detective assigned to collect the evidence was lying prostrate on the floor having fainted and collapsed in a heap. He must have missed lunch.

What do normal people do on a Saturday afternoon? Play sport or go shopping? Take a walk through the woods or by the canal with their kids. Perhaps stay in bed with a lover? Not me. I wouldn't be anywhere but this ill-equipped operating theatre in a district general hospital surrounded by dedicated medical professionals. That said, several of them were already on the verge of a panic attack and I had barely begun the surgery. I was relaxed because I loved operating and this was unusual. A challenging case not routine boring surgery. Did I think about the patient as a fellow human being? What would be the point of that? This victim didn't need an anxious, empathetic surgeon. She needed an effective technician. A Formula one mechanic, not a well-meaning apprentice from the garage on the corner.

I put a blade of the dissecting scissors through the stab wound and slit open the pericardium from top to bottom. Blood clot slithered out into the wound and, with every heart contraction, blood pissed out of the stab wound in the distended right ventricle. What's more, I calmly stood back and let the hole spray like a fountain. This left Wendy Wu somewhat perplexed and visibly frightened the nurses. Had the policeman remained on his feet he may well have arrested me.

'Why are you doing that?' she gasped, suppressing the term psychopath.

THE TRAUMA CHRONICLES

'Look at the heart,' I said. 'How do you expect me to stitch that fragile muscle when it's blown up like a bloody balloon! She's over-transfused. The pressure was low because of tamponade. Look at it now.'

The trace on the screen showed 130/70 and the heart rate had fallen below 100 beats per minute. The wound edges were oozing blood again. Once satisfied that I had let out enough volume to minimise tension, I simply put my finger over the hole and asked for a nylon stitch.

For those who had never seen a beautiful beating heart, let alone tried to stitch a moving target, this was pretty dramatic stuff. But for me it was my day job. I may still have been a trainee, but I had a supreme confidence in my own ability that comes with a modicum of experience and significant head trauma. As Mary Shepherd liked to joke, I walked the fine line between a spectacular surgical career and a prison sentence.

I used three single nylon stitches to close the rent, each carefully spaced and gently tied without too much tension. The sharp needle provoked a run of fast heart rhythm but it settled spontaneously. The defibrillator was not needed. There was a separate stab wound to the right of the breast bone through into the space around the right lung, so I opened what we call the pleural cavity from my midline incision. Air and blood slopped out and into the discard sucker. We didn't have the equipment to recycle and give it back so it was wasted. One of our senior Harefield anaesthetists would have used the discarded blood to feed the roses in his garden.

The pink spongy lung was still oozing blood and air but stitching the delicate tissue just tears more holes. It's like trying to sew jelly. Instead I used the electrocautery to

20

burn and seal the leaking edges. A suction tube drain left in the cavity would evacuate the rest. For good measure I opened into the left chest and sucked out blood from there too. Until that point I had resisted entering into the belly for one good reason. Had the knife penetrated bowel the whole abdominal cavity could be contaminated with faeces and I really didn't want crap to spill anywhere else. So I first covered the chest incision with iodine soaked packs.

Sure enough, there were deep penetrating wounds at various points where the letter T was carved into her. I was curious why he did that—I naturally assumed a homicidal maniac would be a man, with apologies to the gender equality folk. Having stabbed her in the heart, which could be considered a fatal blow, this further mutilation had to be the work of a malevolent psychopath, not a benevolent one like me.

Taking the lid off my next present, there were separate wounds to the liver, spleen and bowel. They each oozed blood benignly but there was no significant haemorrhage that the cautery couldn't stem. In those days we simply used to remove a damaged spleen without understanding the lasting immunological consequences. Clamp the artery and vein, chop through, tie them off and lift it out. Simple. There was a discrete, deeply penetrating wound to the body of the liver, but nature's own clotting mechanisms had sealed that off. I inspected the hole carefully but neither blood nor bile was leaking from it.

That left the more serious issue of the lacerated colon leaking faeces. Again it was a discrete stab wound of 2 centimetres in width. With the windpipe still to repair I didn't want to overcomplicate matters, so I just sewed it up. Purists might argue that I should have protected the repair by creating a colostomy to divert the faeces externally into a bag, but I didn't. I just figured that we wouldn't be feeding her for several days and what bowel contents she still had would pass.

The neck wound turned out to be really scary and, by then, I was becoming restless and irritable. Not physically tired, but annoyed by not having a familiar team and having to ask for every single instrument. Tired of waiting for stuff to be brought from the store cupboard. Tired of explaining to my surgical assistant with initiative failure the help I so desperately needed when he obviously wanted to be somewhere else. And frustrated by Wendy's inability to either push the blood pressure up or ease it down again.

Now for the really nasty twist. Not only had the knife cut through the windpipe but it had also lacerated its immediate neighbour, the gullet. Stomach contents and acid had regurgitated into the wound and spilled over into the airways. Having extended my incision up into the neck, the whole catastrophe was there to see. The right jugular vein had been severed too but that didn't matter much. It had clotted under finger pressure courtesy of the ambulance man who likely saved the woman's life. I mused that I should let him know that, but her survival was not a foregone conclusion at this stage. With the body cavities split wide open, the scene resembled an autopsy, not a delicate operation.

By now I felt the need to be nice to everyone, so awful was the grim afternoon for those less obsessed with multiple stab wounds. Had the policeman recovered yet? He'd been carried out and deposited on a chair with a cup of tea, the British remedy for everything. So I got on and ligated both ends of the severed jugular. She didn't need it.

Other veins would take over by draining blood from her brain. Nor was the windpipe a problem. I closed the tube with simple stitches rendering it air tight again. The gullet is simply a muscular pipe but, given the regurgitation of acid, it was important to keep her stomach empty. We have flexible plastic tubes for that. Patients undergoing abdominal surgery have them passed through their noses and can be fed through them without swallowing. I hoped that if I just stitched the defect and kept her 'nil by mouth' for a couple of weeks it would heal. But I decided to leave the skin and subcutaneous tissues wide open to help prevent infection. Otherwise we risked abscess formation over the repair. Deep, contaminated wounds usually end up filled with pus.

It took another half hour to re-inspect the injuries and insert the drainage tubes. Now that Wendy had dealt with the metabolic mayhem in the bloodstream, the wounded heart was beating away happily. I asked the anaesthetic nurse how much blood the woman had been transfused and was shocked to learn it was twenty-one units. Inevitably, much of that had pissed back out through the stab wounds then down the sucker, but overall her haemoglobin level was acceptable. Having anticipated that Wycombe would not have wire stitches on stainless steel needles to close the breast bone, I had sent a message to Harefield theatres requesting them to dispatch some. Needless to say they hadn't arrived by the time I was ready for them so I took a bladder break. No Lord Brock's operating boots this time.

As I cast off sweaty rubber gloves and blood-soaked gown, Wendy caught a glimpse of the dark patch of sweat down the back of my shirt.

'I see you're human then' she said. 'I was beginning to wonder. You seemed to be made of ice.'

A barbed retort came quickly to mind. 'I am made of ice but it's too warm in this theatre. I'm melting. I'll be back when the wires arrive.'

My new friend Wendy Wu looked concerned. 'Don't leave me for too long,' she bleated, with an unexpected air of insecurity from someone who had brilliantly kept the butchered woman alive for three hours. Then the obvious dawned on me. Two strangers had rapidly bonded as a team in an attempt to save a young life. It was the stuff of medical soap operas. The reason so many surgeons find themselves in the divorce courts.

I ambled back to the accident department and out onto the ambulance deck, craving fresh air in the late Spring afternoon. The blood spattered reception bay had been cleaned. It was now occupied by a groaning cyclist with a broken arm. No one seemed to be interested in him, including myself. It had rained but the sun was now shining and the walking wounded were trickling in from their sports fields. A collection of muddy, bloody knees and bandaged heads reminiscent of my own rugby days in Cambridge. A little old lady with a limp asked me to help her to the reception desk which I was delighted to do. As she sat on a bench to begin the endless wait she thanked me and enquired how long I had been a porter there?

'Feels like forever,' I said.

There were no mobile phones in 1980 so I needed to check in with the Harefield switchboard. But as soon as I lifted the receiver those wire sutures arrived by taxi at reception so my thoughts were diverted. Wendy was pleased to see me back.

'She's been stable,' she exclaimed with an air of disbelief.

'Why should she not be?' I responded, as if wounded by the remark. 'I've stopped the bleeding, and hopefully you've backed off filling her with cold fluid. And the bastard that tried to kill her will avoid a murder charge. Hopefully she'll make it now, poor woman. You had better warn intensive care that she'll be with them shortly.'

I didn't verbalise my obvious concern. Who would take over her care when I rode off into the sunset? The repair job was only the start. Besides wistful Wendy Wu, the silent surgical registrar, and the wibbly wobbly policeman no one else had shown a blind bit of interest in the case.

After a final, self-congratulatory inspection of the happy heart and its neat stitches, I rammed the stainless steel wires through each side of the breast bone. You can't tie knots in wire. It's a matter of tightly twisting them together until the bone edges are firmly opposed, then snipping the ends off with wire cutters. By then I'd had enough. I asked the fading registrar to shove the guts back in the belly and sew up the rest of the gaping wound. Then he should let his boss in the clubhouse know what we had done.

Wendy Wu dropped her mask and smiled at me as I stepped back from the operating table. Between us, we had pulled off a dramatic rescue without a blazing political row as to who was in charge. It had been a gallant team effort between the gentle consultant anaesthetist and a belligerent trainee cardiac surgeon. For the first time in hours, an air of solace and contentment descended upon theatre 2.

There followed a bout of pure 1980s surgical theatre as my adrenaline rush was replaced by testosterone. First, I sat quietly in a corner and wrote the operation note. Drawing all the wounds, recording their depth, and describing the damage to the underlying organs. If we had indeed avoided an autopsy, my writing and illustrations would become an important legal document. At the same time, I was watching Wendy gathering her equipment together and sauntered over as she was preparing the move to intensive care. By this point in the proceedings she was very attractive to me. It's a hospital thing, the interest that emerges if the chemistry is right. The mixing of acid with alkali in the test tube that is the operating theatre. Shake them together and the fizz pours over the top.

'Are you from Hong Kong?' I asked Wendy as an opening gambit.

'Yes I am' she replied. 'How did you guess that?'

I could have said your eyes gave it away but I had learned not to be too personal with Chinese women. So I simply said 'I've just been operating in Hong Kong for a couple of months. I love the place.'

That broke the ice, and it transpired that her father was an anaesthetist at the University Hospital. Perhaps I had met him there, but that wasn't the point. I was on the verge of asking her to have a drink with me that evening when a nurse interrupted.

'Mr Westaby, there's a phone call for you in the corridor. Its Harefield Hospital I think they said.'

Oh bugger, I thought to myself, but I just murmured 'thank you.'

On the Road Again

Do not go gentle into that good night – rage, rage
against the dying of the light.

Dylan Thomas

The switchboard girls all called me by my first name.

'Steve, your senior house office asked us to find you. One of Mr Jackson's post-op patients had a cardiac arrest half an hour ago. They managed to get him back and take him to ITU but they need you to come and look at him. They think he's got a chest full of blood.'

I didn't say anything for a while. The profound 'oh shit' moment paralysed my tongue. Not because I wanted to make out with Wendy, though the idea had crossed my mind. On the contrary, it was my responsibility to see our attempted homicide patient settled in the intensive care unit before starting back to headquarters. Yet, Harefield was where I was meant to be when they needed me. Could they call Mr Jackson himself? That's not how things worked in those days. I could hear the blip blip blip of the portable monitor as Wendy and a theatre porter pushed the bed through the swing doors. She could see I was crest fallen.

'Wendy I'm afraid I have to go and leave you to it. I'm really sorry.'

Was I fooling myself or did she look disappointed? What she said lingered with me for the rest of the weekend.

'Ice man, you were great. Come back when you can. I wanted to hear about your adventures on my island. Another time maybe.'

Perhaps that call had prevented me from making a fool of myself. Again.

It was 6.30 pm in the evening as I turned into the nearest garage to fill my petrol tank. As I drove back down the A40 towards London, Kiss FM radio were playing Christopher Cross 'Ride like the wind' and I was certainly pushing it speed wise. The blatant misdemeanour reminded me that the police had asked to interview me after the case. I guess my interest in Wendy had pushed that to the back of my mind, and in any case it was too late now. Should they still want to ask me stuff they knew where to find me.

In Harefield, the village pubs were packed with cheerful folk sitting out by the roadside. Lots of hospital staff were amongst them but, as the saying goes, there's no rest for the wicked. The house officer who summoned me back was already downing a pint of beer in the mansion bar when I pulled him back to intensive care. They were expecting another cardiac transplant later that night and were not terribly happy about an unexpected emergency admission from the wards on an understaffed weekend.

I knew the patient well enough. He was an affable chap in his seventies, a lifelong smoker who had undergone removal of part of his gullet for cancer earlier in the week. No one knew why he had suddenly suffered a cardiac arrest but, with a history of angina,

ON THE ROAD AGAIN

I suspected he'd had an undiagnosed heart attack during the operation. That could have caused a sudden rhythm disturbance during the afternoon, followed by a period of external cardiac massage, then electrical defibrillation by the duty resuscitation team. A follow up chest X-ray showed at least a litre of fluid around the left lung which the juniors had interpreted as blood. But he wasn't shocked. Instead he looked flushed in the face and was warm not cold. I had that sinking feeling about it when I spotted bubbles of air behind the heart shadow.

'What do you think is going on here?' I enquired of the house officer.

'I think we've probably broken a few ribs with the cardiac massage and he's had a bleed from the incision.'

'Doubt it,' I responded. 'Look at the gas here. It wasn't there on his previous X-ray.' I knew precisely what had happened but thought I should keep my junior colleague in suspense until I could insert a chest drain and remove the fluid collection. I tried to give the lad a clue.

'What did they have for lunch on the ward today? You're usually scavenging for left overs in the kitchen aren't you?'

'Not today,' came the reply somewhat indignantly.

The poor patient looked dreadfully uncomfortable by now, groaning in pain and clutching the left side of his chest so it was time to do something to help. I asked his nurse to bring a wide bore chest drain and vials of local anaesthetic. Frankly, besides a lumbar puncture with a sharp needle probing within millimetres of my spinal cord, the worse thing I could imagine was having a chest drain shoved between the ribs within centimetres of the heart. To avoid excruciating pain it has to be done well. Lots of local anaesthetic, then a scalpel incision all the way through the chest wall. The plastic tube with its sharp metal introducer can then be slipped in without resistance.

So many times had I watched the novices make tentative scalpel incisions then ram the metal road agonisingly—and in vain—against sensitive ribs. On one occasion, a junior colleague shoved far too hard and the drain shot directly through into the main chamber of the heart. When he removed the introducer, bright red blood pulsed out. On that occasion, a clamp on the tube and a rapid chest incision saved the day. Others have not fared as well with chest drains entering the lung, or passing through the diaphragm into the liver or bowel.

There was no such drama this time, but my fears for the man were justified. Stomach contents hosed out into the plastic tube. That lunch time, the patient had taken his first solid food since his operation. Either the surgical repair gave way then or perhaps later during the external cardiac massage. Stomach acid burning away the sensitive lining of his chest cavity accounted for his agony, but now wasn't the time to re-operate on him. We needed to drain the fluid and hydrate him with an intravenous drip until he was fitter. Did I mind if he was moved back to the ward, given their shortage of staff overnight for the transplant? I thought that was unreasonable. Why add risk for one patient when the other hadn't even reached the hospital yet? That's what I argued but I knew I'd be overridden. Should I invite my boss to join the dispute at 9 p.m. in the evening? Not a bit of it. In any case, it would make no difference. The transplant juggernaut rumbled on whatever else took precedent. That's the way it was.

ON THE ROAD AGAIN

At least one thing cheered me up. 'Peanut child' had woken up from the anaesthetic, had a coughing fit and expectorated the fragments I had abandoned. He had gone home happily during the early evening with a clear chest and grateful parents. I was hungry and dehydrated myself but, without setting off into the village again, beer and crisps at the residents' bar was my only option. Perhaps the other surgical residents would be there before they embarked on the transplant donor run. Otherwise I would settle for an ancient leather armchair in the television room with metal springs sticking into my backside. I'm sure it belonged to Billyard-Leake. But my rear end wasn't to be sore for long. When the bar phone rang I hoped it was to tell the transplant boys to get out on the road. It wasn't. Despite the crackling on the line across the room, I heard them ask for me.

My spirits took a dive as dismal possibilities came to mind. Perhaps the patient in Wycombe was in trouble, or the leaking stomach patient had gone back to the ward and arrested again. Inevitably, it was something grim at night when switchboard were chasing me.

The night operator was a good friend by now. Frank had been sympathetically calling me out for months.

'Hello Frank. Is it bad news or worse tonight?'

There was a dearth of his usual cheerful banter.

'Don't expect you want to hear this on a Saturday night, Steve, but I have Barnet General on the line. They want to discuss a patient with you.'

I sighed audibly and he picked up quickly on my irritation.

'I'm sorry, I've heard you've had a tough day already, but at least you're not involved in the transplant. The

THE TRAUMA CHRONICLES

donor is in Nottingham and they're meant to be going by car.'

'Agreed' I said. 'Put them through then, Frank, let's find out what's happening in Barnet tonight.'

'Hello Sir, are you the thoracic surgeon on call? I wonder if you could help me.'

This was the polite lilt of an experienced orthopaedic surgeon who had just assessed a road traffic accident victim in their accident department. The patient was a male motorcyclist with multiple injuries sustained during a high speed collision with an articulated lorry on the A1 dual carriageway. So far, their investigations had revealed displaced fractures of the spine and pelvis and he was semi-conscious with a head injury. Listening to the chest there were reduced breath sounds on the left side and the X-ray showed fluid, presumably blood, in the space around the lung. *So far, so what*, I said to myself. *Just put a bloody drain in the chest and see what comes out. I'm not going to provide a continuous itinerant chest drainage service for the whole region.*

The softly spoken orthopaedic surgeon finally came to the point.

'My main worry on the X-ray is the widened mediastinum.'

The mediastinum is the central part of the chest between the lungs which contains the important anatomical structures therein–the heart, the main blood vessels as they emerge from the heart, then the windpipe, gullet and a lot of lymph glands. The sinister significance of a 'widened mediastinum' in road accidents is that the biggest artery in the body, the aorta, can tear during abrupt deceleration. The heavy column of blood in the aorta reverberates like a bell clanger and the rip occurs at the point at the back of the chest where the vessel is tethered by its branches to the spinal column. Many patients bleed out immediately or before reaching hospital. A few survive when their injuries cause an abrupt fall in blood pressure and blood clot under the lining of the chest prevents exsanguination – much like the stab wound lady earlier that afternoon.

A spinal fracture with bleeding from the bone can present a similar X-ray appearance. So I asked him 'what level is the spinal fracture? Is it in the chest?' It wasn't. It was in a lumbar vertebra behind the abdomen. The lower spine and pelvis had probably been shattered when the motorcyclist hit the barrier in the central reservation. No, it was definitely the upper part of the mediastinum that was widened. Should we both be proven correct in our expectation, the young man needed emergency surgery to repair that huge vessel as soon as it could be arranged. So I set my beer down on the floor next to the chair. One last question.

'What is his blood pressure now?'

'It's around 100/60 after a couple of litres of dextrose-saline. We're waiting for some group O blood.'

'Please don't push it up any higher,' I responded. 'If you do he'll rupture. I'll set off now. Can you ask the theatres to get their thoracotomy set laid out?' I sincerely hoped that they had the right equipment. This was going to be a very high risk operation for this tired trainee.

One vital piece of equipment I anticipated their hospital wouldn't have was the type of special vascular clamp that works best in the chest. Not that I had ever repaired a ruptured aorta on my own, but there had to be a first time for everything. So I wandered past theatres to pick up the necessary instruments before setting off. They were busy preparing for the night's activities, expecting the donor heart to arrive in the early hours. Would I prefer to transfer a ruptured aorta to Harefield and operate with nurses and an anaesthetist I knew? Certainly, but there was no chance of that. In any case his orthopaedic injuries needed careful attention too. Barnet General was one of Mary Shepherd's far flung outposts which she kept to herself. I had never been there before and, setting off in the dark, it occurred to me that I didn't even know where Barnet was, never mind the hospital. Just as there were no mobile phones in those days, the Sat Nav hadn't been invented. So I reluctantly pulled over under a lamppost in the village to study a map of North London. It looked like I should head to Watford, take the A41 then follow the signposts.

That chest X-ray was straight out of the text books. The widened superior mediastinum was barn door obvious with some free blood in the left chest. Despite the blood loss, these patients develop high blood pressure because the body's biological sensors are pushed away from the lumen of the aorta by clots in the tissues. Artificially registering low blood pressure, those receptors cause reflex constriction of the smaller blood vessels to raise it again. The result – soaring blood pressure, then free rupture of the torn vessel with rapid exsanguination. What was the lad's pressure now, 150/90? Shit and derision.

The orthopaedic surgeon, Ismail, had the on call consultant anaesthetist and an operating theatre team standing by for us, but with two appendix operations, a strangulated hernia and an abscess on the bum already waiting, they didn't want to waste time.

ON THE ROAD AGAIN

'Let's get him up there and asleep,' I said. 'The anaesthetic drugs will bring his pressure down. Then I'll need him in the left lateral position. How stable is the spinal fracture?'

Unstable spinal fractures were always a worry, and ideally would be dealt with before anything else. Turning the man on his side risked displacing the bone fragments causing compression and injury to the nervous system. I had good reason to be considering that. A selfish reason, to be honest. Putting clamps across the damaged aorta completely cuts off blood flow to the lower half of the body including the spinal cord. Because of that the repair would be critically time dependent. Should the clamps remain in place for more than thirty minutes, the lack of blood supply could result in paraplegia. Alternatively, he might be paraplegic from the fracture already, in which case I didn't want to be blamed for it.

'Do you know whether he's moved his legs?' I asked Ismail.

'No I don't,' was his response. 'He's not really been conscious or cooperating since he came in. There's a tense bruise over his left temple where he banged his head, but the last time I looked his pupils were still equally sized and reacting to light.'

In other words, no information. In 1980, there were no CT or MRI scans so opinions based on clinical experience really mattered. And that is how we gained our experience in those days. By taking responsibility and standing proud at the operating table. I had seen an attempted traumatic rupture repair once before with Miss Shepherd. It was distinctly scary and a bloody disaster. She was clearly uncomfortable operating on the

THE TRAUMA CHRONICLES

aorta and lost control. The patient bled to death over both of us. But now it was my turn.

There was an old adage in surgery—see one, do one, teach one—which is now obsolete. Why? Because in the contemporary era of reporting surgeons' death rates in the media trainees are not allowed to engage in anything that might risk their boss's reputation. These days, no trainee will operate on a transected aorta. So when they encounter their first case as a consultant surgeon they will be in the same position as I was. The death I had witnessed was weeks before, but now I was going to attempt to fix the dreaded problem myself in an unfamiliar environment with a team who would rather not be there on a Saturday night. Just like Wycombe, none of them had clapped eyes on me before. The best news was that enthusiastic Ismail was volunteering to be my first assistant and his registrar would hold the sucker in readiness in case everything went 'tits up' and blood sprayed the operating lights.

Was I nervous about the risk of losing the patient in a sea of blood? Not at all. It might happen but that's not what I was expecting. I was already relishing the prospect of telling my colleagues that I had successfully repaired a traumatic ruptured aorta. I was oblivious to fear from the professional standpoint. Was that normal? Absolutely not. Most surgeons don't have the luxury of being disinhibited by a blow to the head.

Between us, we gently positioned the patient lying on his right side, left arm pulled up above his head so I could open the chest between the fourth and fifth ribs. I needed to be directly on top of this injury not struggling to reach it from below. At the same time we were as careful as we possibly could be not to displace

36

the spinal and pelvic fractures. As we painted and draped the broken body our anaesthetist was fixated upon the spectacular bruise on the side of his head. I asked again whether the pupils were of equal size. That was difficult to ascertain given the position with drips and drapes in the way, but he thought so.

It was the second large incision of the day, this time a long cut along the side of the chest from breast bone at the front to spine at the rear. He was a slim, muscular patient and smoke billowed from the electrocautery as it sliced through muscle.

'Can you turn it down a bit?' I exclaimed. 'We're not electing a pope.'

As soon as we breached the chest cavity blood spilled out down my gown and onto the floor. I expected it and cautiously extended the opening between the ribs. In went Harefield's metal retractor enabling me to crank open the chest so the 'dog could see the rabbit.' There followed a familiar crack as one gave way under the strain. Not an issue. I would routinely cut through a rib at the back of the incision in planned operations, but there were no rib cutters at Barnet.

Standing in front of the patient, Ismail retracted the spongy pink lung towards himself. The move exposed a frightening expanse of black blood clot that had spread extensively under the thin, membranous lining of the chest. But that's what saved his life. A similar tamponading mechanism to the stab wound to the heart in the morning. Nature has its own way of dealing with bleeding, but all too often the misguided attempts to normalise blood pressure precipitate fatal haemorrhage before the surgeon gets his chance. When pre-hospital care took precedent over 'scoop and run', the chances of reaching an operating theatre with a serious blood vessel injury declined. I was destined to crusade on that issue later in my career.

The key was not to disturb that blood clot over the top of the injury, but to find short lengths of normal aorta proximal and distal to the tear that could be safely clamped. That involves dissecting blindly alongside the obscured windpipe and gullet, between which are vital nerves and blood vessels that mustn't be damaged. Ismail nervously shuffled from foot to foot as I scraped away lumps of clot well proximal to the tear. Once I could feel the aortic wall I gently advanced a flexed finger beneath and around the pulsating tube followed by a linen tape. Now I had control of the vessel, so when the time came I could clamp it. But first I had to achieve the same beyond the site of injury where the branches to the ribs and spine emerged. If clumsy or unfortunate, it was easy to avulse one of these and cause further bleeding.

Concentration overrides fatigue; at least it does most of the time. It was midnight in Barnet and the pubs had closed. While normal folk were going to sleep, I was thinking *what size tube do I need to replace this aorta?* Everything needed to be in place before I clamped it and began working against the clock.

My plan was simple. Apply both clamps, expose and cut out the damaged segment, then sew in the tube of Dacron to replace it. Straightforward in theory, perhaps. Less so in practice. At rest the aorta carries five litres of blood around the body each minute. The sewing had to be blood tight and achieved within a time frame that would not leave him paralysed below the waist and

ON THE ROAD AGAIN

incontinent. Hence my concern that the spinal trauma could have rendered him paraplegic already.

With my instruments in hand, the phrase 'ready, steady, go' came to mind. Clamps applied cautiously across the aorta, above and below the tear – two minutes. Blood clot scraped away from the damaged tube – another two minutes. Inspection of the tear and surrounding aorta – two minutes, and so it progressed as the spinal cord pleaded for its blood supply back. I chopped out five centimetres of the traumatised vessel and took the equivalent length of Dacron tube to replace it. These obsessional anastomoses, as the joins are called, take time and concentration. At least five to ten minutes each, so there is absolutely no room for error. Operating in a cardiac centre with a heart-lung machine to cool and protect the nervous system can provide the luxury of more time. But not in Barnet General where it was 'shit or bust'.

As I tied the last knot with the graft in place the process had taken twenty-seven minutes with the clamps in place. That was gratifyingly fast for a first attempt. As I released the clamps the circulation for the lower half of the body was restored and blood pulsed around the vital organs again. There was oozing through the stitch holes and a couple of spurters that needed an extra stitch but no need to clamp again. Ismail sighed in relief. The registrar went out to relieve himself. I suspected that he'd had a few beers before we started.

In self-congratulatory mode I put in two chest drains and began the tedious process of closing up. Once the ribs were approximated and the first layer of muscle closed, Ismail dispensed with the seniority issue and kindly offered to finish off. Frankly, I was knackered and didn't need to be asked twice. It was ten minutes to two and a cheerful auxiliary nurse brought me a cup of coffee. 'You deserve that' she said and I wasn't about to dispute it. It felt a very long time since I was searching for peanuts.

Between us, we carefully repositioned the man on his back and I asked the diligent anaesthetist to lift the eyelids and check the pupils. He did so, hesitated for a moment, and found a brighter light to look again. The pregnant pause told the story. The pupil in the right eye, the opposite side from the large bruise over the skull, was dilated and didn't constrict. A blown pupil signifies brain compression beneath the site of the injury. What's more, I didn't need to be a brain surgeon to know what that meant. It was a fundamental issue in trauma that we learned about in medical school. Bleeding within the skull was now compressing the brain with pressure on the nerves to the eyes. Eventually, tension within the rigid box pushes the lower brain through the base of the skull causing breathing to stop, then death.

Reviewing the events of the evening, it was the classical presentation for a cerebral haemorrhage or subdural haematoma as we call it. He was unconscious when the ambulance picked him up by the roadside. Then he came round with a lucid period during which he was able to describe what happened to him. But, by the time Ismail and his team saw him in the accident department he was undoubtedly drowsy again, smelled of alcohol and vomited. When they asked him to move his legs there was no response. After the chest X-ray proved worrying, the aorta became the focus of their attention and they didn't ask for skull films. So he could well have a fracture beneath that swelling.

ON THE ROAD AGAIN

What were the options? Despair and say 'we tried our best' in which cased my own gallant efforts were wasted. Or call for a brain surgeon from one of the regional centres? They would just say 'transfer the patient' but there was no time for that. It was 02.30 a.m. and he was deteriorating fast. That left me with a conundrum. Should I get on and do it myself? That's what I told Ismail we should do. Trephining the skull for blood had been done by military surgeons for hundreds of years. What could be difficult about it?

I asked the theatre nurses whether they had a drill and bit in the cupboard somewhere. I was keeping my fingers crossed that the patient had an extradural haematoma—a collection of blood between the damaged bone and its fibrous lining, not within the brain itself. Without modern imaging, any attempt to locate the problem was a fishing expedition, a bit like drilling for oil. And from my surgical exams, I knew that simple brain swelling and bleeds deeper within the skull were more common than the issue I was banking upon. But an extradural bleed was the only diagnosis we could reasonably treat and if we didn't intervene he was definitely going to die. So I didn't have the vaguest reservation about doing it.

With his head positioned with the bruising uppermost, I asked the nurses to shave off the matted hair. Beneath was a tell-tale laceration which I extended surgically to expose the bone. There, much to my satisfaction, was a skull fracture. More a cracked eggshell than a shattered bone but it was testimony to the severity of the blow. By then, a World War II brain surgery kit was neatly laid out beside me on blue drapes. I had seen similar in the Hunterian Museum at the Royal College of Surgeons

41

but it still took me a while to work out what I was looking at.

To begin with, we attached an arrow shaped perforator to the drill bit and I set about excavating the bone. This ground out a conical shaped hole until the point just penetrated the inner table of the skull. No blood yet. The next step employed a blunt ended rose burr to excavate a cylindrical tunnel through the full thickness of the bone. That causes the marrow to ooze blood, but congratulations Barnet General, you even had bone wax on the set to control it. So far my tentative exploration hadn't hit on the extradural collection I was hoping for. The last move was to incise the membrane between bone and brain with a sharply pointed scalpel blade. Still no cigar.

Ismail wasn't too disappointed by that. He dealt with trauma on a day to day basis and appreciated that it might need several attempts at different sites to locate the offending clot. So I tried again a few centimetres behind the first hole. Perforator, rose burr, scalpel, more frustration. I was feeling like an offending clot myself. Yet the ominous fact that the heart rate was slowing and the blood pressure spontaneously rising without transfusion told me that we had to continue. If this was just brain swelling he was doomed anyway. Should we locate bleeding beneath the fracture, he had a chance of recovery.

I drilled again, this time further forward above his ear. Perforator, burr, but I didn't need the blade. Blood gushed out of the tunnel and onto my clogs. Had that happened during the aortic repair I would have been truly pissed off. Blood pouring over me from the skull – happy days. Ismail and his registrar cheered spontaneously, more like a football match than an operating theatre in the middle of the night. Fortunately, the drainage slowed then stopped in little more than a minute. Then both the blood pressure and heart rate drifted down. On this pitch it was Westaby 2, Grim Reaper 0. At least it was at that point.

Once more, my Barnet boss told me to step down and allow the home team to finish. This time, the kindly nurse returned with coffee and a chocolate biscuit while I wrote the operation notes. Like most NHS facilities for staff, the rest room was a drab and dismal place with worn chairs, strip lights and torn curtains. Green curtains. The message was clear. We don't want you lot sitting around relaxing even in the middle of the night. Get on with the next case. For once, I hoped that my day was finished. Sixteen hours of adrenaline-fuelled concentration and physical endeavour eventually takes its toll. That is why it was me on the road not Mr Jackson or Miss Shepherd. Trauma is a young man's sport.

Suspicious Minds

Our greatest weakness lies in giving up. The most
certain way to succeed is always to try just one
more time.

Thomas Edison

I had a lover. Or at least I thought I had. Like everything
else in life, bar surgery, I neglected her, which she didn't
deserve. It goes without saying that we met in a hospital.
She was Sister McDougall from the accident department
in Cambridge, where I would strut my stuff or end up with
my own injuries on a Saturday evening after rugby. Sarah
was a free spirit who grew up by Kenya's lake Nakuru
before training as a nurse at the Middlesex Hospital in the
West End. Stark contrasts. Her father was one of 'the few.'
A Battle of Britain spitfire pilot who, on hearing about
me, counselled her sternly against unprincipled hospital
Romeos. But she cleaned my wounds, stitched my torn
scalp and injected antibiotics after I fractured my jaw.

The two of us worked side by side, resuscitating
patients in shock and relieving others in pain. That's
what brings doctors and nurses together in a way that
other professions can't. I was iron filings to her magnet,
but not alone in that.

The woman was stunning and everyone knew it. She
stood 5ft 9ins in her nurse's shoes, a 21-inch waist,
jet black hair and a face like an angel. I ruined my

own marriage then her existing relationship through indiscretion. Then when I left for London with just a suitcase, Sarah followed. I had created havoc in her life.

Now, in the Emergency Department at the Royal Free Hospital she was known as Sister Beautiful, widely admired for her nursing skill, looks and compassion. But, just as I did, she returned alone at night to her single room—or cell being a more accurate term— in the nurse's home. Harefield was many miles from Hampstead. Hong Kong had been even further. And she was fully aware that the following year I would head off alone to train in the United States.

Sarah knew that she couldn't afford to give up her job and come with me. Did we have a future together? I certainly hoped so, but my ruthless ambition rendered any personal life as difficult as it could be. Sitting alone and exhausted in the dismal surgeons' room that Saturday night, I started to think about her. Sarah would understand what I had achieved that day. She had cared for damaged brains, ruptured aortas and stab wounds to the heart, many of whom did not survive. Like a schoolboy cricketer who hit his first six, I wanted to share my day with her. I wondered why I treated her so badly. Not a sensible thing to do to a famously attractive woman. The teaching hospital nurse surrounded by type A personality males. Doctors, medical students, paramedics, not to mention the many patients who drooled over her. I had witnessed it all for myself in Cambridge but, shamefully, I hadn't yet visited her at the Royal Free.

By then we were both so busy that we didn't meet very often. It had been weeks since I last saw her. She had been bright and bubbly as always. Energised by being back in London where she trained. I liked to listen to her stories from the front line and the arse end of life. She cared for tramps, politicians and drug addicts alike, treating them all with the same kindness and respect. The previous week, she had tried to save the victim of a cold blooded assassination attempt. The man had been shot at close range through the head and was expected to die. But she spurred on the resuscitation team to work hard and give him a chance. When they walked away it was left to Sarah to treat him with respect.

The case turned out to be headline news in London the next day and, for once, she had something to counter my continuously egotistical dialogue. It became a murder investigation, with police swarming around the department, wanting to interview her. *Who would not want to interview her?* I thought. What's more, she admitted that she rather fancied the detective in charge. She had teased me with that and I hadn't heard from her since. Only now, in the dead of night, did I take that seriously and it didn't sound funny anymore.

It occurred to me, in the gloom of the dreary sitting room, that Barnet was only fifteen minutes from Hampstead given empty roads at night. On the schedule she kept me up to date with, it said she was working nights this weekend and I figured that at 4 am the department might be quiet. I had an urge to see her and wondered about calling in by surprise. I mused that I might entice her out to the car for a grope given the mood I was in. Then again, Saturday nights in the Emergency Department were always busy with drunks and drug addicts. Perhaps it would be a wasted trip and leave me stranded in Central London when I should be back in Harefield. So I decided to call first. Theatre rest room phone to Barnet Hospital switchboard. Switchboard to the Royal Free Hospital, then please put me through to the Emergency Department.

A female voice answered.

'Good morning, could I speak with Sister in Charge?' I said.

'Yes, but I know she's busy at the moment. Let me see if I can find her.' The handset was set down and I could hear continuous hustle and bustle in the background. They sounded so busy that I was relieved to have called before making the journey. I was also excited in anticipation. Almost wetting myself to hear her voice again. I pictured her in that starched blue uniform, with silver belt buckle, white cap on curly black hair, piercing blue eyes and endless legs in black stockings. Miss World in a swimsuit simply didn't compare.

Then an unexpected twist.

'It's Sister Jenkins. Can I help?'

It was one of Sarah's friends whom I had met on a couple of occasions. Given that there was only one sister on at a time at night I was immediately confused. After a pause I replied, 'Oh Jenny, its Steve Westaby. I wasn't expecting you. Sarah told me that she was doing the nights this weekend.' In the midst of a frantic shift Jenny responded without thinking.

'No, she did a swap with me last week. She said she was going out tonight. I assumed she was with you. Sorry but I need to get back to the guy I'm stitching up. His head's full of glass.'

'Ok' I responded dejectedly. 'Do me a favour and don't mention that I called in the middle of the night, will you. Bye.'

My long day had taken a turn for the worst. I suspect that I looked crestfallen as Ismail ambled in, grinning broadly.

'We're all closed up and that blown pupil has come down. They're almost equal again.'

The praise was almost irrelevant now. Dejection had caused me to feel particularly weary, and the sudden mistrust of my wayward lover took precedent over triumphalism.

You might consider that saving a life is a marvellous thing, but I was constantly buggering up my own. I had the distinct image of my lover sleeping soundly with someone else in the early hours of the morning. If so it was unlikely to be in the nurses home. The beds were too small and I was sure Sarah would command a better offer. So no point drifting down there to knock on the door. Moreover that wouldn't be fair. She surely deserved a better life than she had with me.

'Looks like the long day has caught up with you,' murmured my new friend.

'I guess it has' I replied. 'Any blood in the drains?'

'No all's good. He's stable now.'

We discussed whether it was the right thing for Ismail to go on and operate on the broken bones. I didn't think so. The patient had had four hours of surgery to his head and chest and his body temperature had fallen in the meantime. I felt that a prolonged period of stability in their intensive care unit under a warming blanket was more important than fixing his skeleton. Ismail agreed. We would turn off the anaesthetic and move him to a bed. You can never be sure about the brain. We had decompressed it, but recovery was still unpredictable. Further orthopaedic surgery was futile unless he woke up and demonstrated the propensity to survive.

Having aced out with the Royal Free I had to call the Harefield switchboard and catch up on the weekend. For all they knew I could be in a night club in the West End by now. But I soon wished I hadn't bothered. My good friend the night time telephonist had been waiting to pass on a message. There was an unstable case in the intensive care unit in the Central Middlesex Hospital that they wanted to offload to us as soon as possible. No further information. Despite the fact it was 04.30 I asked to be put through to my junior, the resident registrar on call who was obliged to remain in the hospital. Or at least in the mansion bar, as was the custom in those days. He didn't respond. A nurse answered his bleep for him at theatre reception. The transplant wasn't going well and the lad had been summoned to help. So I asked to be put through to intensive care and was very polite to the nurse who answered.

'Hi it's Steve. I've been asked if we can accept a patient who may well need surgery in the morning,' which it was already. I didn't have the opportunity to say more, nor was I asked what was wrong with the patient. If I had been I would have had to confess to not knowing. 'Not a chance,' came the response. 'Your Registrar was trying to get us to take back Mr Jackson's case. Apparently he's not doing well on the ward but we're full. Sorry.' At least she was sympathetic and it was not fair to get aggressive with her.

Now I was left completely up in the air. It was a balancing act. I really didn't think I could contribute much more to the man at Harefield leaking acid into his chest. Neither myself nor Mr Jackson could get into an operating theatre to improve matters, even if that were the right thing. Nor would he have access to an intensive care bed afterwards. The chest drains were his best chance, but someone needed to sort out whether they were blocked with food debris from his stomach. I left a message for the registrar to look into it when he re-appeared from theatre. Failing that, for an intensive care nurse to wander up to the ward and check during her break. Now I had to deal with the Central Middlesex.

An abundance of adrenaline and testosterone usually kept me ablaze at times like this, but losing track of Sarah had somewhat doused the flames. I was beginning to fade. Worse than that, my vivid imagination left me troubled and distracted. This cocky arrogant prat of a surgeon had taken his much admired nursing sister for granted too often. I had worried about that in Hong Kong. We just never saw each other anymore and I foolishly expected this wonderful woman to toil in her pressurised environment then hibernate in the nurses home until I turned up again.

After a couple of abortive attempts I finally get through to the Central Middlesex switchboard. But by now, I'm a little abrupt. 'It's the chest surgeon from Harefield. I understand you've been trying to get hold of me.' The response was polite and efficient. 'I'm putting you through to intensive care now, Sir.' Disarmed by the pleasant reception, I wound down a gear, at least for a few seconds. Then I got 'ITU, sorry we're very busy, can you hold the line for a minute?' For a moment all my frustration, fatigue and personal jealousy spewed out and I revved up again. 'No I fucking can't. It's the thoracic senior registrar from Harefield. Do you want me or don't you'?

I immediately regretted the expletive. It was my prospective patient that they were exercised by, needless to say. So the poor nurse apologised profusely and muttered 'Sorry. I'll get the doctor.' It was a young trainee surgeon called Phil who came to the phone. A switched on Guy's graduate I knew from my time as a registrar at the Hammersmith Hospital. I could trust his judgement so at least that was a good start. What's more, he sounded relieved to have a familiar voice on the phone.

'Steve I've been looking for you. Harefield told me you were on call and I need some help here.' I was immediately tempted to ask where's his consultant was, but I held back on the confrontational stuff. The answer came without enquiring. As was frequently the case in that era, one specialist was covering two hospitals and he was apparently embroiled in action at 'St Elsewheres'. Trauma rarely took priority.

Phil's patient had been found groaning on the bonnet of his car on London's North Circular road following a head on collision in the early hours. The impact propelled him through the windscreen. There was no compulsory seat belt legislation in 1980, and we were both familiar with the patterns of injury that unrestrained drivers suffered. The chest and abdomen always smashed against the steering wheel and the face or forehead hit the dashboard. The combination of head, chest and abdominal injuries occurred frequently, but most hospitals only had general surgeons so they did what they knew best. Open the abdomen to take a look. I had little choice but to set off down the A1 freeway and across North London to take a look. Bye bye Barnet and on with the next.

52

After hours of disinfectant and diathermy smoke, the fresh early morning air came as a relief. Even with the car windows wound down I found it hard to dispel the enduring odour of burning bone from my nostrils. As I drove west on the North Circular towards Wembley, the sun hauled itself above the horizon behind me casting long shadows on the lamp posts. There was little traffic early on a Sunday. Just a few taxis with inebriated party goers heading home. Was Sister McDougall amongst them? She had every right to be. Then, as the famous football stadium came into view, I saw blue flashing lights and firemen in the distance clearing debris from the road. This was the accident with wrecked vehicles still in place. So smashed that it made me wonder whether there had been fatalities.

I slowed in curiosity and, sure enough, there was the car with a shattered windscreen and streaks of blood on the bonnet. A couple of hours before there had been frenetic activity here with ambulances on scene and police cordoning off the site. Given the state of the second car, the fire brigade must have piled in to cut the passengers out of the wreck. In that era the firm objective was to extricate the injured and take them as quickly as possible to the nearest casualty department, irrespective of the expertise found there. While rapid transit had much to recommend it, salvage from certain death needed skill and expertise. Survival was therefore a matter of Russian Roulette. Sometimes the patient got lucky, more often they didn't. Yet take it or leave it was a part the NHS. Cheap but not so cheerful.

The hospital was close by now. It was next to the Park Royal Brewery in Acton and I could smell the beer already. It was virtually next door to the headquarters of my training rotation—the famous Hammersmith Hospital and Royal Post Graduate Medical School. But they did heart surgery mostly and were far too snooty to entertain a peripatetic practice for chest trauma.

Heading to meet Phil in the intensive care unit, I passed through the Accident and Emergency Department on the way. Out of curiosity I asked the young casualty officer 'were any fatalities brought in from the North Circular crash?'

'How did you know about that?' he replied. 'Actually there were two. Both with fatal head injuries. An unfortunate old couple on their wedding anniversary. A drunk driver wrote them off. He's upstairs in ITU, I believe. Are you the surgeon from Harefield they were looking for?' I assumed he knew the answer to that already as I was still wearing the same theatre blues from Saturday morning. *Property of Harefield Hospital* was embroidered on the shirt pocket to discourage theft, but no one would want mine now.

As I meandered through the dilapidated corridors of this dreary building, I reflected upon the fact that I was here to help someone who had just killed two innocent people on their special day. Doctors are meant to reflect on their practice but I needed to park my feelings on this matter pretty quickly. It wasn't my business to be judgemental. I was there to do the plumbing. Others could take the man to task. Then it occurred to me that I hadn't even learned the names of my first two patients of the day. I just got on and operated on them too. Did what was required and moved on. So this case would be the same.

I needed to press a buzzer to be let into intensive care. Why? Because in those days in London people would wander in off the streets to steal drugs. An expansive West Indian lady in a well filled uniform opened the doors then looked me up and down as if I had just crawled from beneath a stone. I guess I looked like a dishevelled theatre porter at best and they were expecting the patient to go back there. So she said 'you'll have to wait. He's too unstable to move at present.'

I replied in a measured way 'That's why you've dragged me down here from Harefield. I've not come for a night out.'

That embarrassed the poor woman but, as it transpired, there was not much time to waste on pleasantries.

Even at that hour there was a restless crowd faffing around the patient; the tell-tale sign that things were going badly. Phil was relieved to see me at the door and beckoned me across to the bedside. The monitor screen told the story. Blood pressure 60/40 mm Hg, heart rate 130 beats per minute, both registering severe shock. Yet curiously, for a patient with ongoing blood loss, the pressure in the main veins was higher than it should be. For a patient without a penetrating chest wound that was unlikely to be cardiac tamponade.

Phil said 'I'm sorry to bring you down here at this time of night, but as you can see we're losing him and I'm not sure why.'

I was a chest surgeon so my first comment was 'Can you show me his chest X-ray?'

We put it up on the screen at the end of the ward. The black and white picture that always tells the story – for me at least. As I worked through the image methodically I asked my anxious friend why he decided to open the abdomen, and what precisely did he find?

Phil's explanation was that the man was obviously in shock and complaining of pain in the upper abdomen. Because there was bruising and abrasions where the lower chest had impacted on the steering wheel he had been concerned about a ruptured liver or spleen. This was a straightforward and reasonable approach. Several litres of clear fluid and four units of blood had been transfused already but none of it seemed to restore a satisfactory blood pressure. There was a catheter in the bladder but the kidneys were not making urine.

When the belly was opened some fresh blood spilled out but certainly not enough to explain the refractory state of shock. Both spleen and liver seemingly looked undamaged from the midline incision, so Phil closed him up again hoping for the best.

Historically this was the big issue in caring for trauma patients and it persists today. Generalists did what was within their remit but were blind to territory they had not been trained in. Anything above the diaphragm in Phil's case. But all cardiothoracic surgeons had to complete years of general surgical training before moving on to the chest and for the injured patient's benefit that was invaluable. Working with Professor Calne in Cambridge I'd had experience of both liver transplants and liver trauma and I smelled a rat here, so to speak.

That chest X-ray showed three important things that concerned me. First, there was bleeding into the right side of the chest and there had to be at least one litre. Second, what appeared to be the diaphragm on that side was higher than it should be and I suspected I knew the reason for that. But third, and very worryingly, the contour of the heart shadow in the left chest was unusual. The apex of the heart was definitely tipped upwards. Again, I had dealt with enough chest trauma from the Harefield practice to understand what was going on. It explained why the blood pressure in the arteries was low but the pressure in the main veins was elevated. It wasn't simply due to over transfusion as was usually the case.

While we were talking about the X-ray appearances away from the bed, the agitated anaesthetist called us back.

'We're losing him!'

She was right about that. With the blood pressure dipping to 50 mm Hg she was squeezing the blood bag to force more fluid into the circulation as fast as she could. But it wasn't helping, so I asked her to hold off for a while.

'Do you have an emergency chest opening kit?' I asked the nurse in charge of the unit.

'We have some instruments, yes. But you're not going to operate on him here are you?'

My response was a bit mean but I was weary and irascible. 'It's your choice. Do we stop now and let him go, in which case I'm leaving? Or do you want me to make some sort of effort? If so, get us the bloody instruments and a gown and some gloves.'

The poor chap went pale with chastisement and set about doing what I asked. Would I have snapped at a woman like that? I doubt it, but what I said did the trick. There was clearly no time to bring an operating theatre team back into the hospital to set up for a chest operation that they were wholly unfamiliar with. As it happened, there wasn't even time to wheel him back down the corridor to the theatre doors.

'He's arresting,' screamed our frantic anaesthetist.

The response to cardiac arrest is protocol-driven in every hospital. A junior doctor with crossed palms pumps rhythmically on the breast bone squeezing the heart against the spine. That substitutes for the lost cardiac contractions. At the same time the anaesthetist blows oxygen into the lungs through the tube in the windpipe. The well tried process works when the pumping chambers are filling passively between cardiac compressions but that was not the case here. What's more, the heart itself hadn't even changed rhythm. It was deprived of oxygen because the blood pressure was low but hadn't fibrillated yet. It had not reached the stage, often reproduced on the television, when the defibrillator goes *zap* and the patient elevates from the bed through spasm of the 'erector spinae' back muscles. So I told them to stop the pumping because it wouldn't do any good. They should shoot a bolus of adrenaline into the drip instead.

Within seconds, the heart rate and blood pressure increased sufficiently to buy time. Without wasting the minutes taken to scrub up, I pulled on a sterile gown and gloves and told Phil to do the same.

'What are we aiming to do?' he bleated in bewildered fashion.

My brief retort was 'you'll see in a minute. Just help me will you.'

I needed to make our hesitant anaesthetic colleague aware of my intentions. She was a trainee, too. Moreover, it was increasingly apparent that she was way out of her depth and ready to piss her pants.

'Don't you have a consultant to back you up?' I asked.

'I called him soon after the patient arrived. He just said "carry on and do your best." It's always the same at weekends. But when you tell me what you want I'll do it.'

Trying his best to help now, and expecting me to open the chest, the charge nurse asked whether I needed the man rolled onto his side. But which side? I had an evolving strategy in mind but I hadn't explained it yet. In the era prior to scanners the key to effective trauma surgery was simply to predict the injuries from the patient's history and plain X-ray findings. Pure detective work. 'Clinical acumen' is the profession's phrase for it, yet nothing beats experience. Having spent many hours in an Emergency room in New York's Harlem, after leaving medical school, I'd had a good start.

Having viewed the crash site on the way to the Central Middlesex, my thoughts on what had happened to the man had crystallised somewhat. It was a high speed collision which wrecked both cars and he had not been wearing a seat belt. His chest and upper abdomen would have been driven hard against the steering wheel. Bruising on his skin suggested that and there was a pattern of injury that goes along with it. The abdominal contents were pressurised acutely and forced upwards. That's what smashes the liver and ruptures the diaphragm. Part or all of the liver herniates through into the right chest then bleeds into the space around the lung. Phil had interpreted the chest X-ray appearance as showing the diaphragm pushed upwards by blood below it. But I could also see multiple rib fractures on the picture. Broken ribs are painful and the nerves beneath them supply the abdominal wall. So the patient has what we call 'referred pain' in the belly which can be mistaken for damage to the internal organs. Yet it was even more complicated than that. I suspected that the upper surface of the liver was torn, which Phil would have missed from below. So blood filled the chest not the abdomen. Detective work not rocket science.

Given that the man had received copious amounts of intravenous blood and fluid, why did his blood pressure not respond predictably by going up again? I suspected that the answer lay with a rare injury that would soon kill him. I had encountered it just once before in the autopsy room, and if we were going to intervene it had to be quickly. Worryingly, I was going to have to carve open both sides of the chest on an intensive care bed without either operating theatre lights or nursing team. We were a 'rag, tag and bobtail' group of tired and hungry trainees, earnestly attempting to salvage a homicidal maniac in circumstances not fit for veterinary surgery.

I told the charge nurse to scrub and hand the instruments to us. I urged our trembling anaesthetist to park her panic attack and just hand ventilate the lungs and asked for someone to please phone switchboard and bring in the operating theatre staff. Should he survive and need closing up again, we would need lots of stuff that was not available on the emergency instrument set.

Mental and physical fatigue are two different things. Sure I was weary after a straight twenty-four hours at the coal face, but tiredness was never an excuse for anything in those days. Cardiac surgical trainees were not allowed weaknesses. We were the special forces of the medical profession and the adrenaline rush during emergencies more than compensated for lack of sleep. Yet there was barely time to prep the skin and put on drapes. Phil was securing the folded edges of the linen to the man's skin when we heard the words 'he's arresting

SUSPICIOUS MINDS

again.' I needed to gain access to his heart in the left chest while lining up the cut so I could continue it across the midline into the right side. We called that a 'bucket handle incision' which was used in the early days of heart surgery before a saw was developed to bisect the breastbone.

As I hacked through fat and muscle it was only reasonable to warn the onlookers that the process would be gruesome. One positive at this point. Dead people don't bleed.

'I'm going to need the retractor in a second, then you'll see what the problem is,' I said confidently, implying that I had exclusive insight into the cause of his demise. Then I murmured to Phil 'have you worked it out yet?'

With more cutting between the fourth and fifth ribs the chest cavity was breached. A modest amount of blood spewed out onto the white bed sheets and, as we cranked open a window, there was the left lung. When I pulled that aside my suspicions were confirmed. Instead of seeing the grey fibrous pericardium that encapsulates the heart, we were staring directly upon the quivering muscular pumping chambers, the right and left ventricles, doing not very much at all. This was a ruptured pericardial sac with herniation of the ventricles caused on impact of the steering wheel against the breastbone. The dislocated heart suddenly becomes strangulated between the collecting and pumping chambers. That explained why the pressure in the obstructed veins draining into the heart was high and the blood pressure low. What's more there was obvious bruising in the battered muscle of the right ventricle from the catastrophic impact. That was why the large

61

volumes of transfused fluid could not resuscitate him. Only surgery could sort this out.

My instinct was to put my fist around the ventricles and perform open chest cardiac massage. Yet that could not help until I had relieved the strangulation. My gawping assistant seemed mesmerised at the sight. So I told him 'Just keep that lung out of the way while I enlarge the tear, Phil.'

He was clearly fascinated by the process, which was good, but distracted from any initiative needed to be useful. I knew that those obstructed atria would be distended and fragile, so I decided to open up the pericardium away from the site of rupture. Then I could cut down carefully into the tear. I was working against time with no circulation to his brain though the heart so far had maintained its normal rhythm. Should it lose electrical coordination did they have internal defibrillating paddles in the hospital? The question produced a sea of blank faces which meant 'we don't know.'

I couldn't see within the pericardium and sure enough the tip of the scissors perforated the tense right atrium so that blood gushed out. I felt an anxious flutter of my own heart at that point. There followed a series of expletives and a rushed attempt to complete my intended manoeuvre. Fortunately that did the trick. It was like removing a noose from the heart's neck. The deprived ventricles filled with blood and the pressure in the atria dropped precipitously. As a result, the bleeding from the perforation slowed to a trickle. I was tempted to start internal cardiac massage right then but was concerned that the physical assault might cause the heart to fibrillate. So I asked for another slug of intravenous adrenaline instead. There was just enough flow remaining to trickle the hormone into the coronary arteries and, once it reached the feeble muscle, the heart took off like a train.

For the first time since the crash, this drunk driver had an unobstructed circulation with an adequate blood pressure but we needed to ensure that continued. Like a spent Jack-in-the-Box, I needed to replace the dislocated heart back where it belonged then with a couple of widely spaced stitches, stop it from jumping out again. It took longer to find suitable stitches than to insert them, so the tedium of 'amateur night' was beginning to wear thin.

In the face of renewed stability I had choices to make. The irritated operating theatre team had returned and arrived in intensive care to see who had the temerity to call them back. So would it be better to proceed in exploring the right chest leaning uncomfortably over the bedside without suitable lights? Or should we close the left chest, having dealt with the disaster, and take him to better working conditions in the operating theatre. It was a no-brainer and fortunately Phil, the home player, agreed with me.

Diplomatically I thanked the astonished theatre nurses for coming. They stood silently, gawping at the huge hole in the patient's chest until I told them that I needed to do the same on the other side. I got an inordinately stupid reply. 'We don't do chest surgery here.' I said 'well you do now, so let's get moving shall we. He's still bleeding.'

That wasn't a flippant remark, it was purely factual. Despite his much-improved circulation, the blood pressure had started to drift down again. Phil asked where I thought he was bleeding from.

THE TRAUMA CHRONICLES

'He's got a torn liver that's filling the chest through a ruptured diaphragm,' I said, confidently but consistent with having succeeded with the immediately life-threatening problem. 'It's the dome of the liver that's damaged which is why you couldn't see it from below.'

Feeling somewhat non-plussed at this point he just said 'Oh.'

The anaesthetist, whose name I still didn't know, was happier and readily cooperative. So the circus moved on to its next venue. The clock on the wall said 07.45 and it occurred to me that I had been wearing the same theatre clothes and wallowing in blood for twenty-four hours. What's more, given some down time, I began to feel jaded. I wasn't alone in that. Phil and the anaesthetist had also been working all weekend, day and night. It's what we did.

While Phil helped the nurses get the patient into position for the right thoracotomy, I turned on the shower in the surgeons' changing room, discarded my sweaty uniform and let cold water splash over my head.

At times like this, cold showers usually succeeded in reviving me to the point where I could function again. The high density of cold receptors in the skin bombard the brain with electrical impulses which instantly increase alertness, clarity and energy levels. This happens through the abrupt release of endorphins as the body struggles to maintain its core temperature. Cold also ameliorates stress by boosting antioxidants in the blood, so when I walked back into that operating theatre I was in a better state to perform than the rest of the crew. It was Sunday. A new day. Another twenty-four hours on call.

It Gets Difficult

> I regard the brain as a computer which will stop
> working when its components fail. There is no
> heaven or afterlife for broken computers. That is a
> fairy story for people who are afraid of the dark.
>
> Stephen Hawking

A pulped liver protruding through a split diaphragm is a truly awesome sight. At least it is when you eventually see it after scooping blood clot out of the chest. Happily, the patient's own clotting mechanism together with low blood pressure had stopped most of the bleeding, which is why he had survived to this point. As you might imagine, you can't stitch liver as you can other tissues. I avulsed fragmented pieces with my fingertips. Oozing edges I cauterised with the diathermy, and one significantly sized bile duct I attempted to close with a stitch. But ultimately, the safest thing is to cover what remains with linen packs, close up, then remove them a day or two later when nature has succeeded in fixing its own problem. I learned that in Cambridge. Dreaming spires in the city, desperate battles in the hospital.

I enjoyed pushing the swollen organ back down through the diaphragm and into the abdomen where it belonged. Having succeeded, I then set about stitching the torn edges together with the packs beneath. Positive pressure inflation of the lungs by the ventilator would help keep everything in place and, crucially, Phil was aware how many packs we had left in situ. When the time came to retrieve them he could do that through his abdominal incision. I didn't anticipate coming back to the Central Middlesex for that pleasure.

The vital signs remained stable during the course of the procedure, and our charming anaesthetist had said so little that I thought she may have fallen asleep. But when I did eventually ask her how he was getting on the news wasn't encouraging. She was giving more transfusion because the blood pressure was sagging again and the thing that concerned me most was the trauma to the heart itself. It looked battered and bruised. It had been crushed between breast bone and spine and, as well as contused muscle, there could be structural damage inside that we didn't know about.

In similar circumstances, I had seen thrombosed coronary arteries with myocardial infarction, torn heart valves and traumatic holes between the pumping chambers. So I asked whether anyone had listened to his chest with a stethoscope. Was there a heart murmur? Blank faces, though I could hardly blame them when I hadn't done it for myself. Should there be another problem, what could I do about it? Nothing. There was no heart-lung machine in this district general hospital. Nor could I arrange to transfer him to Harefield with no intensive care beds. We had done our best. Heart problem or not he would live or die right here. Those poor souls he collided with were in mortuary fridges already. Did I care whether he lived or died? Of course I did. He probably had a loving wife and kids at home. How must they feel?

IT GETS DIFFICULT

Phil offered to buy me Sunday breakfast in the canteen while Acton and normal people came to life. Of course, hospital breakfasts are just about as unhealthy as you can possibly imagine but the fried bread, eggs, bacon and black pudding were just what I needed. Sitting there, it occurred to me that I hadn't eaten a meal since the previous morning. Over lousy coffee we caught up on each other's careers since moving on from the Hammersmith. Then he asked probingly about the lovely nursing sister he used to see me with.

'Wasn't Sarah her name? Are you still going out with her?'

I remembered that Phil used to chat her up in the doctor's mess while she waited for me to extricate myself from the cardiac operating theatres. I always knew he had an interest in her so I was rather mischievous.

'Not any more,' I said. 'She got pissed off with the fact that I was still married.' Phil's eyes lit up in the gloom.

'Oh, I'm sorry to hear that.' Which he wasn't! 'I don't suppose you have a number for her do you?' I lied again.

'I'm afraid not. She was working at the Royal Free but I think she's gone back to Africa. Her family is still out there.'

Though my report card would read *must try harder*, I wondered about calling the nurses' home but decided against it. Did I really want to find out that she wasn't there? What I really needed to do at this point was to call Harefield and report in.

So far it was a quiet Sunday morning. Mr Jackson's leaking oesophagectomy case was septic and on antibiotics. He would either improve sufficiently to be operated on again, or most likely not. Another hospital was trying to have us admit a breathless patient with a chest full of pus, but that would have to wait. I had seen enough of the Central Middlesex for now but Phil wanted me to take a last look in intensive care. I'd already told him 'once I've gone he's all yours. I'll be operating all day Monday.'

There was still a crowd around the bed sorting out the various drips and drains. The nurses didn't handle many chest drains in the unit, so when I said 'don't forget to put them on suction' they didn't know what I meant. Did they have a system to suck on the underwater seal? 'Don't know.' Exasperated already, I told Phil to sort it out and make sure that they didn't just attach powerful wall suction to the tubes. That would drag the lungs out of the chest.

Where was the nice anaesthetist whose name I missed? She had gone to bed already. Having attached the patient to the ventilator and issued instructions to keep him asleep, she signed off at top speed. It was a new day. He was someone else's problem now, though no one was certain whose that might be. There didn't seem to be any bleeding through the drains but his blood pressure had sagged further to below 100 mg Hg. Nor was there any urine in the catheter from his bladder. Liquid gold we call it, and when it stops flowing after shock it means that the kidneys have shut down. Tedious but only to be expected. I assumed that they could arrange dialysis if he needed it.

It was then that I asked his name and looked at his face for the first time. It was smashed horribly from colliding with the dashboard and shredded by windscreen glass. If spared, he would need a faciomaxillary surgeon but I had a gut feeling that he wouldn't get that far. I said as much to my colleague, who now had the unenviable task of caring for a killer.

IT GETS DIFFICULT

'Why?' Phil asked. The response was direct.

'Because his heart is buggered.' I said. 'If you had smashed it for six with a cricket bat it couldn't be worse off. This is what blunt cardiac trauma does. You saw that the right ventricle was bruised. Like tenderised steak. The ventricular septum must look the same.'

I slipped a hand under the sheets to feel a leg. It was cold. After all our efforts he was still in a low cardiac output state, so I signed off.

'Just turn the adrenaline up and see if he responds. Good to see you, Phil. Let me know how things go.' I remembered thinking *it doesn't matter what that face looks like at the crematorium. I hope he doesn't have children.*

This time, I slipped on my seat belt for the drive out of town in the sunshine. The roads were quiet and I wished for there to be no chest injuries in the whole region that day. Let alone to myself. Yet I still had the compulsion to let rip in the old MG and get some wind in my hair. So instead of turning off the A40 back to Harefield I opted to continue northward to High Wycombe to see yesterday's patient. I guess I was hoping to find Wendy in the intensive care unit too.

The speedometer hit 95 mph as I passed the overpass at Beaconsfield. My head was in the clouds and I failed to register the police vehicle waiting for idiots to fall into their speed trap. I was almost at the Wycombe turn off by the time I heard the siren and spotted the blue lights flashing in my rear view mirror. What's more, I knew what to expect as it wasn't the first time. I could almost recite their opening banter as I pulled over.

With a supercilious smirk on his face, one of the officers ambled slowly from his car to mine. He stopped to peer through my open window and, after a good look around, asked 'why are you still in your pyjamas at this time of the morning Sir? Have you been to a sleepover?'

I was tempted to tell him to 'f*** off' but had learned through bitter experience to avoid unnecessary conflict with the law. So I respond politely 'take another look officer. I may have been wearing these clothes all night but they are surgical scrubs not pyjamas. And I'm speeding for good reason. I expect you heard of the attempted homicide yesterday. I'm the surgeon from Harefield who operated on the poor woman. She's not doing well and I'm trying to avoid a murder case. That becomes more likely every minute I sit here, however much I'm enjoying your company.'

The glib expression on the cops face was priceless as he carefully pondered over what to say next. Fortunately for me it was a charitable response. First he asked to see my driving licence, which I truthfully said was in the wallet in my jacket in the surgeon's changing room at Harefield. They were welcome to turn around and go look for it. Then he said 'Ok Sir, let's get moving. We'll escort you into the hospital so you don't get into any more trouble. Stick close behind and we'll put the blue lights on.' And so it was that I had a police escort through the town and to the doors of the casualty department. They weren't stupid. I'm certain that they wanted to be sure of what I'd just told them.

I was happier about the journey than I was about the patient. She still looked deathly pale as if she'd had an autopsy. The incisions in her chest and belly were now respectfully hidden beneath adhesive dressings and white linen bed sheets. But, despite the pallor, she had a raised temperature with rapid heart rate and sagging blood pressure. Her nurse volunteered that she had been stable overnight and the doctors were pleased with her progress. The blood pressure had only dropped in the last hour and there hadn't been any urine in the bladder catheter during that time.

'What are they doing about that?' I asked. 'Is Wendy around?'

I wasn't sure whether I was asking that for my own benefit or the patient's. She'd been in first thing in the morning and had been happy. Not since. My aspirations for Sunday lunch in a pub with her were now fading.

I could see the reason for the fast heart rate and low blood pressure on the monitor.

'How long has she been in atrial fibrillation?' I asked. Blank face. 'Has anyone done anything about it?' The poor girl was clearly flustered and embarrassed by the fact that an intensive care unit had not registered the change in heart rhythm. Especially when the drop in blood flow had already caused the kidneys to pack up.

'I'll call the doctor,' was the only thing she could find to say. I clearly looked irritated and intimidating, which was unintentional but perhaps not surprising given my extended day. When the junior doctor arrived ten minutes later I was more direct.

'What do you make of her condition right now? Are you happy with it? Do you have anything to tell me?'

The young man, who did not speak good English, was disarmed by an unexpected full frontal assault on a Sunday morning. But let's be clear about the consequences. This potential homicide patient was deteriorating unnecessarily through lack of informed care. I performed the surgery and would be held

71

responsible. Nor did I have the option of transferring the poor woman to the Harefield intensive care unit, so it was just as well that I had turned up. Atrial fibrillation is common after any surgery on the heart and should be dealt with promptly. So I told him that we must shock the heart back into a normal rhythm right now. The woman was still unconscious so we didn't need an anaesthetist. Just find the defibrillating paddles and get them to the bedside.

Before zapping her I needed to see the blood test results from the morning. Sure enough, the blood biochemistry was deranged and needed adjusting before shooting a bolt of electricity across her chest. But I didn't have all day. I syringed a vial of potassium into her circulation myself and connected the external defibrillating paddles to the machine. I asked the house doctor to set the output to 50 Joules but he was still flustered and unsure as to what to do. Not the calibre of medic you need with you in an emergency. The nurse did it for him and I smeared grease over the chest to prevent burning. I placed one paddle firmly over my midline incision through the breast bone and the other in the left armpit. Then pushed the button and *zap*.

As sudden muscle spasm elevated her frail body from the mattress I stared intently at the monitor screen. The electrocardiogram looked like a scene from the Dolomites. Jagged squiggles of ventricular fibrillation, with squirming, purposeless muscle achieving nothing. No problem. I half expected it. I simply instructed my dysfunctional assistant to recharge the machine to deliver 100 Joules. Then zapped again. This time a flat line with no electrical activity. Dead heart, but nothing I couldn't handle. A thump directly over the heart caused it to contract once in response. Another whack produced a run of electrical complexes, then a pause.

I quietly asked the nurse to give me a hypodermic syringe and vial of adrenaline from the resuscitation trolley because I was reluctant to launch into external cardiac massage and disrupt my wired-up sternum. I shot the adrenaline into the drip in the neck and thumped the chest again. The resulting electrical activity was sufficient to pump the stimulant into the heart's blood supply and it responded gratefully. We had succeeded in establishing normal heart rhythm again with blood flow to the brain. Adrenaline certainly cheers up a flagging heart but it has a downside too. It clamps down the small blood vessels and shoots up the blood pressure making it harder for the heart to pump. As dramatic as all this might seem, stopping and starting hearts was my day job and would be for the next forty years.

Having dealt with the immediate problem, I tried to formulate a care plan with what staff I could muster. They comprised the patient's nurse, the sister in charge of the unit that day, and the hapless junior doctor who had little to contribute. First question, 'who exactly is going to take responsibility for the case?' As a visiting trainee surgeon that couldn't be me. Sister didn't know. That would have to be decided on Monday. Somewhat indignant after all my efforts, I threw in a line of my own, 'that's if the patient survives the weekend.'

She had a raised temperature already and, following deep stab wounds from a dirty kitchen knife, sepsis was an ever present threat. In those days, as now, it was not advisable to dish out hefty doses of antibiotics without good reason. Given the fever following wounds to both heart and gut, I asked that they send blood samples to the bacteriology laboratory for culture. Then, how long were they intending to keep those chest drains in place? Was anything still coming out into the bottles? No. So as another potential conduit for infection, they should be removed. Disillusioned by their efforts, I decided to do that myself. It was the best way to signify that my role had reached its conclusion.

Signing off in frustration, I suggested that they withdraw the sedative drugs so hopefully she would wake up and breathe for herself. Then they could remove her from the ventilator and withdraw the tube from her injured windpipe. It was important to cough and clear her airways, but remember—no food or fluid by mouth through the repaired gullet. That needed a couple of weeks to heal and they needed a surgeon to take responsibility for that. Thankfully, sister was taking notes but nothing was going to get done over the weekend. It was time to leave and that was the last time I saw the poor woman. Did she have family waiting anxiously at home for her? I daren't ask. That was just too upsetting for me to contemplate.

As I pulled up by the main entrance at Harefield in broad daylight, there was a fox rummaging around the rubbish bins. I sat silently for a few minutes watching it. Not something to be seen at transplant centres like Stanford University, Groote Schuur, or the Mayo Clinic. It was an NHS thing.

Harefield wasn't a happy place that morning as the transplant hadn't gone well. Mr Jackson's patient had died from sepsis overnight and switchboard had been trying to track me down for more than an hour. Again, I had that sinking feeling, but unnecessarily as it happened. The duty registrar just wanted to talk to me about some potential referrals for which we had no beds. More chests full of pus and cancers obstructing the windpipe. The usual thoracic surgery emergencies. All I could say was what we always said, 'sorry the beds are full at the moment we'll let you know when things change.' The NHS has always been that way.

I was knackered now. Perhaps it would have been sensible to have debriefed with someone about the night's cases but I was beyond that. I needed a nap for a couple of hours then hopefully a wind down with a few beers in the village pub that evening. The standard surgical coping mechanism.

Bright sunlight shone through my huge third floor mansion windows with their vista over the lake and valley beyond. While content with the night's work, I could picture my two year old daughter playing in her garden near Cambridge and felt infinitely sad. I wanted to be with her in the sunshine. Bouncing her on dad's knee or pushing her on the swing. Instead, she barely knew me. I was just another grown up who turned up from time to time to be berated for spoiling her with gifts or sweets. Fortunately, a lapse into unconscious spared me from further pain at that point, just in time to abort my agonising about leaving for America at the end of the year. Ambitious father, bloody useless dad, sad character, summed it up.

All too soon the dreaded phone rang and shattered my peace in the late afternoon. I deliberately ignored it at first, but then my hospital pager went off with the message to call switchboard. The operator, Elaine, sounded relieved to get a response.

'Steve, I've got Hemel Hempstead Hospital holding on the line for you. The doctor sounds really anxious.

THE TRAUMA CHRONICLES

Can I put her through?' I grunted in tacit agreement. What else could I do even if I was sinking with exhaustion now?

'Is that the thoracic surgeon?'

'Yes it is. What can I do for you?'

'We've got a terrible problem here in casualty at Hemel. An awful transfixion injury. The boy was playing on scaffolding for a new office block and apparently fell from the third storey. He's got a pole passing straight through the left chest and his head and neck are swollen. The fire brigade cut him free but he's in shock and it's so close to his heart. Can you come please?'

'How old is he?' I asked.

'Just twelve,' came the reply. 'He's very distressed.'

Who wouldn't be, I thought. I looked at the alarm clock on the bedside cabinet next to the phone. It read twenty past five.

'I'll be there by six,' I said. 'Can you move him up to the operating theatre and cross match six units of blood?'

'We have to order it from St Albans,' came the reply.

'Then get the police to bring it across' I said. 'We're going to need it in theatre before I open him.' I realised that the last statement sounded a bit as if he were a can of beans. For the second time that weekend, I left Harefield like a bat out of hell.

In contrast to my morning escapade, I had a genuine reason to put my foot down. Did I know how to get there? Roughly. Head west towards Watford then northward on the M1 motorway. At Hemel, ask directions to the hospital. I had never been there before. For that matter, I had never encountered a 'through and through' transfixion injury either and was energised by

76

IT GETS DIFFICULT

the prospect of having to deal with it. But I honestly did not want to meet the poor boy while he was still awake. I anticipated that he would have been put to sleep and be on a ventilator by the time I arrived. But no. They were afraid to take that step given an air leak from his bronchial tubes that was inflating his head and chest like the Michelin Man.

Horror movies paled in comparison with the reality of the scene. He was lying on his right side, still fully clothed. The metal scaffolding tube protruded from the front and rear of his chest for at least twelve inches and both his shirt and the stretcher were soaked in bright red blood. Though heavily sedated, he was still whimpering pathetically. Beside him, his poor parents were holding on for dear life. The weeping mum was cradling his head. Dad clasped onto a cold sweaty arm, supporting it as the shoulder blade grated against the pole in his back.

The boy's pallid, swollen face and puffy eyes were testament to a serious lung injury. What's more, the blood had made its way up the windpipe and was spattered around his nostrils, yet to the tutored eye the fact that he was still alive showed that the heart and major blood vessels were intact. Nor had he damaged his spine. Horrific though it seemed at the time, I felt optimistic that we could save the lad. I had no doubt that operating on his chest would be easy enough but it was clearly going to be difficult to find a suitable position to put him to sleep then pass the breathing tube into his windpipe.

I really wanted an experienced anaesthetist this time, with a special endotracheal tube that could close off the left lung while continuing to ventilate the right. I was not going to get that expert help from the home team so

I made a suggestion. If they were agreeable I would ask a paediatric gas man from Harefield to come and help. Hopefully he could bring appropriate equipment for a twelve-year-old. In the meantime, we would spend the waiting time getting him into optimum condition for the surgery.

What could I say to assuage the misery of those despairing parents? They had been surrounded by doctors and nurses in panic mode because chest surgery was way out of bounds for Hemel. But we would help with that so I told them what they wanted to hear. That before long the stake would be gone and the damage repaired. By night fall, they would have their son back. Was I certain of that? Of course not. Would it have helped any of us to discuss the risks of him dying? Not at all. While I sweated away in the operating theatre, some peace of mind for them was worth the gamble.

Needless to say that kindly approach, which I held onto, is not regarded as politically correct. A wish to relieve fear and anxiety was a career-long weakness of mine which has been clobbered out of sight by contemporary risk management in the NHS. To protect the hospital on the medico-legal stage we are supposed to verbalise every risk of a procedure before the consent form is signed. So what ought I report to these poor people? Should I explain that I am not a fully qualified surgeon, just a trainee? Might I offer to call in one of my bosses while warning that they may not arrive before their son bleeds to death? Would it help them to know that I might have to remove a whole lung? Or that the shattered chest cavity might well become infected by the filthy pole? Or that nerves to his diaphragm or voice box may have been severed? Maybe the transfused blood

IT GETS DIFFICULT

was contaminated by hepatitis or AIDS as happened to thousands of other NHS patients. Perhaps the intensive care unit might suffer a power cut so that his ventilator fails. I was never defensive and could never bring myself to do all that stuff.

Chris, my Harefield colleague, came very quickly and together we set about preparing the lad. A slug of barbiturate into the drip rendered him blissfully unconscious. A great kindness at last which allowed us to escort his parents away from the anaesthetic room. Access to his throat to pass the tracheal tube was the major challenge. It was vital not to displace the scaffolding pole in case it was blocking a damaged blood vessel. We didn't have an X-ray, but listening to the chest with a stethoscope there were no breath sounds so it had to be full of blood. The only option was to manhandle the supine body onto the side of the operating table so his right flank was supported on it, with the left chest dangling with the pole in place. Once Chris had safely inserted the tube we rolled him back onto his right side to present the transfixed left chest uppermost for me to operate on. Difficult.

It gave me confidence to be operating with a familiar friend this time, and though visually spectacular I did not expect the surgery itself to be difficult. I had a South African junior doctor as first assistant and, between us, we cut away the blood-soaked clothing and painted his body with iodine. Having fallen backwards, the pole had entered his chest below the shoulder blade then exited through the front above the nipple. Visualising its passage, I was concerned that the root of the lung had been destroyed, hence the brisk air leak from damaged bronchial tubes.

I drew the scalpel blade all the way from the protruding post at the front to the entry wound on his back. Then cut through the muscles of the chest wall down to the ribs with the electrocautery. Three ribs were shattered at the entry point, with bleeding from the arteries beneath. At the exit, the pole had simply dislocated the junctions between bone and cartilage close to the breast bone. No matter. These were the least of my problems.

As I breached the chest cavity, purple blood clot slithered out onto the drapes followed by a splurge of dark blue liquid blood. Air frothed out from the depths confirming an injury to the bronchial tubes so, with renewed urgency, I inserted the metal retractor, spread the ribs, and urged my assistant to suck furiously. Grabbing the offending implement I lifted it away from the lacerated tissues and ceremoniously tossed it onto the tiled floor with a clang. It rolled away noisily before halting under the theatre technician's foot. Not that I noticed. I was frenetically scooping out more blood and clots so I could repair the damage.

Most of the spongy pink lung was collapsed. As I dragged it upwards towards me, the traumatised blood vessels and bronchial tubes came into view so that the extent of the problem became clear. The root of the lung had been torn, with the bronchial tube to the lower lobes being completely detached. With it, the arteries and veins were bleeding but it seemed hopeful that I could save the upper lobe. As I squeezed the hilum to stop the bleeding, I said 'give me a bowel clamp' to the scrub nurse who was eager to please but had never seen a chest operation before. She was clearly bewildered that I asked for a bowel clamp when there were no guts in sight, but none of the chest instruments I would normally use were on her trolley.

With aforesaid instrument in my right hand, I dragged the lung upwards and applied it as close as it would fit to the midline. That stopped both bleeding and air leak with one simple manoeuvre giving us all some breathing space. Somewhat relieved, I turned away from the operating table and went to sit down for a while on a stool, hoping that we had won the war. And that helped to assuage the tension in the room. Somewhere in the real world I could hear church bells ringing for the evening service. God was with me at the time. Get lost Grim Reaper.

The boy's blood pressure was adequate and stable, and the pristine right lung was more than enough to keep him well oxygenated.

'Good job' murmured Chris. 'I hear you've been on the road all weekend.'

'Seems like longer,' I responded with a hint of exhaustion. 'Not sure how much good I've done either. At least we should get this lad through.'

Mentally rested for a few moments, I returned to the table to finish the job. In a contaminated wound there was no point in trying to do something fancy by joining the damaged ends together. That would take time in a shocked and traumatised patient with the real risk of it all becoming infected. So I decided to remove the detached lower lobe allowing the residual lung to grow with him and fill the space.

Having concentrated intently for the life-threatening part of the case, my attention was beginning to wander. That was a common theme. I could thoughtlessly oscillate between hyper-focus and autopilot depending

THE TRAUMA CHRONICLES

upon the demands of an operation. Equally, I could use right or left hand, but usually both, to make surgery easy. My co-dominant cerebral hemispheres worked that way. Awareness in three dimensions was an inherited gift, not that anyone in my family had ever used those skills. Best of all, like the intrepid pioneers of my specialty who sustained prohibitive mortality rates, I was oblivious to self-doubt.

Of the desperate struggles during that weekend, this last operation gave me the most satisfaction. It had been a devastatingly painful experience for both the child and his parents but I sensed that he was safe now. There were still pieces of shattered rib to remove, the chest cavity to be washed out and the ubiquitous drains to insert, but I had the urge to tell them the worst was over. The Hemel anaesthetist, who had stayed with the lad since admission, volunteered to do that. I half considered whether he should take the bloodied pole to show them. On second thoughts it was a crass suggestion, so I kept it to myself. Remarkably enough, Chris also seemed happy.

'I wouldn't have wanted to miss this,' he volunteered. 'Doubt I'll ever see the like again. He's a very lucky boy. A fraction in the wrong direction and he was a gonner.'

I snipped away the bruised and ragged skin from the entry and exit sites, then cheerfully closed up the incision. The clock on the wall had stopped and the sun was setting outside but I had no concept of the time. Though time itself was immaterial, one thing concerned me now. There was no children's intensive care unit in the hospital, so who would care for the lad? It really needed to be Chris and me. We had to stay with him until he was breathing for himself and could be safely taken off the ventilator.

IT GETS DIFFICULT

On the positive side he was young and fit, not a wheezy bronchitic having a lung removed for cancer. If all remained stable over the next couple of hours, we planned to take out the chest drains, wake him up, then remove the tube from his windpipe. But we couldn't afford to delegate that sequence to the inexperienced home team. It wasn't fair to them or the family. Nor could we move him to Harefield. There was little point trying to negotiate that on a Sunday evening. Even if I persuaded them to give me a bed it would mean that the child with a serious chest deformity on Monday's operating list would be cancelled irrespective of the distress to his parents.

What could we do to increase the likelihood of getting the child off the ventilator that night? Keeping him pain free was the crucial factor. And the best way to do that was to inject both the nerves supplying the fractured ribs and surgical incision with local anaesthetic. Buckets of the stuff. He had suffered enough.

Once again, I called Harefield to let them know where to find me. To my surprise switchboard signed off with 'Oh by the way a lady called Sarah was looking for you. We told her you were away dealing with an emergency. Hope that was the right thing.'

'What time was that' I enquired.
'Just an hour ago' came the reply.
'Sorry but what time is it now, I've got no idea'
I responded.
'It's coming up to eight thirty.'

I thought for a moment. She must have returned from an exciting weekend and been tipped off that I was looking for her. Interesting. Paranoia and delirium were creeping in, so I shut down those thought processes.

When I scheduled Monday's operating list I had packed it with cases that I was hoping to operate on myself. For that reason I wanted to get some sleep. Equally, I had no intention of leaving Chris at Hemel on his own so we decided to pass the time with a couple of beers at the local pub. That seemed an infinitely more attractive prospect than a bedside vigil with mournful parents, but there were problems. First, I was still wearing scrubs and second, my wallet was in my jacket at Harefield so I had no money. No matter, Chris would look after me.

My friend sensed that I was fading. Sleep deprivation was a rite of passage for surgical trainees, and who would relinquish the chance to operate solo at night while the boss stayed in bed? Yet despite the machismo there were consequences. I was increasingly restless, irritable and impatient to see my room in the mansion. Fortunately, Chris was determined not to rush the child's progress.

'We should go back and talk with the parents,' he argued, but I was really not in the mood for that. I couldn't take the sycophantic stuff in the state I was in. I didn't need to be thanked emotionally or praised to the heavens for operating. I had a pragmatic approach. Mechanics fix motor cars, I fixed bodies, and derived huge satisfaction from the privilege. That was enough for me.

Given the high mortality rates in the pioneering days of heart surgery, empathy was never at the top of the patients wish list from their surgeon. Most just wanted someone who could get them safely off the operating table. I had learned as much at the Brompton Hospital where, at the bottom of the pile, I was the one dispatched to warn parents of impending doom. That usually meant that the repaired heart would not separate from

IT GETS DIFFICULT

the heart-lung machine and that death was a foregone conclusion. My bosses assiduously avoided the angst and who could blame them? There were no touchy-feely psychologists to debrief us in those days. As trainees, we would find a sympathetic nurse to talk to. Or gyrate with. That was the best form of stress relief back then, and safer than drinking on call.

However irascible I felt, Chris insisted that those devastated parents should have the opportunity to talk with their child's surgeon and ask questions. He was right, of course. Once more they were huddled by the bedside, the weeping mum holding a cold hand under the sheet, dad with his arm clasped around her shoulder. I was destined to spend my whole career intruding in that same tableau but never regretted doing so. I detested death so much and would go to any lengths to prevent it.

In sweaty blues I looked awful and smelled like a pig but the pair still rose reverently to their feet. I told them to sit down again. Their first questions, 'Is he going to live doctor?' I told them what they wanted to hear.

'Yes he is' I said, 'he's a lucky boy.' Those few words prompted a palpable relief of tension so their shoulders dropped visibly and mum started to cry again. While therapeutic for them, it was overly optimistic from me. Many things could go wrong, with infection at the top of the list. But what I told them in their anxious state worked better than a dose of Valium. I felt obliged to mention that the pole had deprived him of half of the left lung but that he wouldn't miss it. The remainder was more than adequate and he would play football again.

The conversation happened to be a diversion. All the while, I was assessing the boy's condition. Though his body temperature had dropped during the surgery, he was warming under a blanket and his cheeks were pink. Heart rate and blood pressure were virtually back to normal and there was no blood in the two chest drains. The chest X-ray taken on his return to the high dependency unit was very reassuring if you ignored the shattered ribs. So, I told Chris and the boy's nurse that I was ready to remove the drains. Once awake they would be a source of distress for him. Yes, it was much sooner than we would normally remove them but I felt it was safer for me to do it now than leave it to someone less experienced the following day. Should air enter the chest cavity accidentally the residual lung would collapse prompting another call out.

The stimulation as I dragged out the first drain woke him abruptly. He started fighting against the breathing machine and the nurse asked whether to sedate him again. Had we been in Harefield with the paediatric intensive care team I would have said yes. But not here. The sooner he was independent of the life support and things that could go wrong, the better. Chris was less certain but he realised I wanted to get away. What he said was 'Ok the tube can come out but I'll stay for a while and make sure his breathing is fine. We don't want things to go tits up now, do we.' The guy was a gentleman. He stayed at the hospital all night long providing the boy pain relief that wouldn't depress his respiratory efforts.

I left Hemel Hempstead at 11.30 p.m. and drove through the gates of Harefield by midnight. The switchboard was next to the main entrance so I called in to announce that I was back. Moreover, I didn't want calls overnight unless it was something desperate in the hospital itself. The region would have to fend for itself.

IT GETS DIFFICULT

'There's just one thing' I was told. 'That lady Sarah called again at 10.30 p.m. She said you could ring her at the flat if you came back before midnight.' I thought about it, but didn't. I'd had enough trauma for one weekend. The mansion and my bed beckoned, but not before a glass of ale in the bar. That pint was a whole weekend's recreation. But I felt as if I had grown six inches through the experience. Only time would tell whether I had achieved anything. Or whether I had lost my lover.

Disappointment

The pessimist sees difficulty in every opportunity.
The optimist sees opportunity in every difficulty.

Winston Churchill

I was up with the lark and making the incision for the first case of the day when Mr Jackson strolled into theatre.

'Morning Steve. How was your weekend?'

I told him that I had been busy around the region dealing with trauma. That was fine, he expected that, but then came the point of the question. He'd already had a general surgeon on the phone from Wycombe complaining about me. Why should that be, after my sterling efforts? Because the chap couldn't find an operation note so he didn't know what I'd done beneath that whole body incision. So where was it? Sleep deprivation apart, I distinctly remembered sitting in the corner of the operating theatre drawing a diagram of the stab wounds, then annotating the injuries and what I had done about them. It was a careful handwritten document with considerable medico-legal implications. What the hell had happened to it?

But what I did not consider reasonable was to begin my working week on the back foot after spinning like a top the whole weekend. I could feel the anger rising and I was not the best at controlling it.

I set the scalpel down on the instrument trolley.

'Sorry, Mr Jackson, but I did write the note, they have clearly lost it. You do the case and I'll go to Wycombe to find it.'

There was silence and deep surprise as I disrobed and paraded out of the operating theatres in a huff. Yet I didn't go to Wycombe. I stormed off to the secretary's office, repeated the note again with the same drawings, then asked that it be faxed through to the surgeon who had made contact earlier that morning. She knew precisely who that was but I didn't ask. At least in my strop I had sufficient insight to hold on to the original this time. After all, I was going to end up in a criminal court explaining my actions sooner or later.

I hadn't slept long and it showed. Despite my protestations to the switchboard, I'd had a 3 a.m. call from the Central Middlesex about bleeding through the chest drains. I had no recollection about what they said or how I responded. After that I was restless, unable to settle again and concerned about life in general. Whether I acknowledged it or not, sleep is a primary biological need like food and water.

Newly acquired information is replayed during deep sleep to consolidate it. Moreover, the brain has a waste disposal system that works best during sleep and insomnia is linked to cerebral decline. Executive functioning—doing the right thing at the right time—depends upon interplay between the brain's complex emotion regulating centre and the part of the brain which governs our actions. When sleep deprived we become hypersensitive to rewards, our emotions are heightened and we start acting irrationally.

DISAPPOINTMENT

Though the science wasn't understood in those days I had just suffered from that process. As surgical trainees we were continuously being judged on temperament with no consideration for the circumstances. So I went back, apologised to the boss, and removed the next lung full of cancer, which gave me no satisfaction at all. Petulant though it might seem, my brain's reward centre was feeling deprived that morning and it showed.

It transpired weeks later that the savvy policeman, who could not recall the findings because he was prostrate on the floor, had thought to take the surgeon's discarded scribblings as evidence. Naturally, he believed there would be a typed version. I had skipped off without discussing the case and the importance of logging the note in the medical records was not readily apparent to him. Reasonably so.

During the afternoon, a call came through to say that the Wycombe patient was septic and did I have any strong opinion about which antibiotic to use. After multiple contaminated wounds with a dirty knife, infection was always on the cards and her fate would be determined largely by which bug had entered her blood stream. Some were more responsive to treatment than others. My first question was 'has Dr Wu seen her today, and if so what does she think?' Answer: 'I don't know Dr Wu. I think she was just doing a locum for the weekend.'

At that point there was only one path I could take, in all conscience. I really had to go back and make an effort to improve matters. Failing that I couldn't see her surviving. And I still knew nothing about her, not even her name. On my operation note I'd left that space blank to fill in at some point in the future. Sometime, maybe never, I suspected. The phrase 'cut and run' was coined for me, yet ultimately she was someone's daughter, or sister, or perhaps a child's mother. She was precious to someone and though she wasn't officially my patient that didn't mean that I shouldn't help.

It was the first time I'd gazed at her face and I was saddened by what I saw. Her name and family circumstances were known by now but I didn't want to know. She was twenty-four and I simply asked whether the police knew who had tried to kill her. The answer was predictable.

'Her partner, and I gather he's been sectioned in a mental hospital.'

Had the poor parents been in to see her?

'Yes and they're obviously devastated.'

The girl's eyes were taped closed, as is usual for unconscious patients in intensive care, but when I stroked her forehead it was hot and sweaty. Had they changed the dressings on the open neck wound? No.

As I withdrew the sticky tape from the gauze and raised the blood caked swabs I could smell pus before I saw it. Revolting green sticky stuff exuded from the depths suggesting a vicious virulent bug called Klebsiella. Surgeons dread that organism. What's more, if it had colonised one site it was likely to infect others too.

I had an important task now. The pus needed to go directly to the laboratory for analysis. The other wounds all needed to be inspected, swabbed and cleaned, then blood samples sent for bacteriological culture. Everything had to be processed immediately, not left overnight because the choice of antibiotic was critical.

The astute young nurse sensed the urgency in my words.

DISAPPOINTMENT

'Shall I fetch you a dressing trolley?' she volunteered. 'Please,' I said, 'and a gown and gloves if you would. I need to do this properly.'

My helper drew the curtains around the bed and pulled back the sheets. Besides the expansive wound coverings the girl wore disposable paper pants, nothing else. On Saturday she was pale and cool, today pink and hot. Her body pulsated visibly so I was sure this was septicaemia. Bugs multiplying in the blood. Hundreds of millions of them, multiplying by the minute.

As I peeled away sticky dressings from the mutilated abdomen her body moved slightly. Not wanting to rouse her I stopped for a minute. When I tried again she squirmed, groaned and managed to prise open one eye lid by detaching the adhesive. She had blue eyes and silky blonde hair still stained by blood. That one piercing eye oscillated in its socket momentarily, then fixed on me. As if to say 'you bastard.'

I couldn't stroke her head with the sterile rubber gloves so I put my face close to hers and whispered 'It's going to be OK. I won't hurt you. We're here to take care of you.' It seemed to register. She closed the eye voluntarily and went still. I hadn't noticed the nurse inject more sedative into the drip so I naively believed that my calming voice had succeeded. No matter. Drugs are always more soothing than words. The eye was taped again and that brief interaction was my only communication with the girl. I hoped that she thought I was kind.

Having succeeded in saving her from the frenzied carnage of cold steel, someone else had to battle the bacteria. Those bugs in her blood were now the main threat and something had to be done that night. So, having re-dressed the wounds I set about trying to locate a senior bacteriologist. That process, as ever, began with a row with the on call laboratory technician who was not prepared to be browbeaten by a doctor from another hospital altogether. I was then put through to the pathology trainee whom I insisted should discuss the case with her consultant at home. Senior doctors protected themselves very well in those days. What did it take to get help for a brutally butchered young woman after an attempted murder and many hours of surgery? My message sequentially to all three was 'she's definitely septic, her blood pressure is falling, and there's no urine in the bag. I want someone to plate out the pus right now, put it under a microscope and have an experienced bacteriologist tell me what bug we're treating.'

When I finally reached the boss I added the stroppy sentence 'if I can't get help soon I'll get the police involved!' I figured that was rude and somewhat petulant on my part, but why not. There's a big difference between grievous bodily harm and murder, and in this case the outcome depended upon many more folk than just the brute wielding the blade.

Before heading back to Harefield for the evening ward round, I returned to her bedside.

'Did you get anywhere?' asked the switched on Australian taking care of her. It was said with typical Aussie candour and an air of resignation that said 'who on earth is going to handle this when you're gone?' No one else regarded the poor kid as their responsibility and who could blame them. Primarily, it was a thoracic surgery case that should be taken care of in a chest hospital, but chest hospitals didn't have Casualty Departments.

DISAPPOINTMENT

Later that evening I received a call from the bacteriologist at Wycombe reporting that the wound infection was caused not by Klebsiella but by an organism called Pseudomonas. A curious name, because there was nothing pseudo about it. Once in the blood stream it was the real thing and pretty damned lethal for a diminutive female with screwed up metabolism. He recommended immediate intravenous infusion of the appropriate antibiotic in high dosage.

'Who else have you told?' I asked. 'I don't work in your hospital so could you please liaise with the intensive care doctors whose job it is to prescribe the drugs. But thanks for letting me know...' I left out the words *the fucking cheerful news*. I didn't want to reveal myself as the belligerent street fighter I was.

Increasingly concerned for the poor woman, I called the Wycombe intensive unit and asked to speak to the sister in charge. Sadly, I expected to get more sense out of her than the junior doctors. What she told me made me miserable. The blood pressure had fallen precipitously since my visit so large doses of adrenaline were being used to support her. Was there any urine coming, the liquid gold of circulatory support? None at all since mid-afternoon and only a trickle all day. Could I have made a difference if I had chained myself to the bedside that Saturday afternoon? Sadly, I considered that a possibility. Heart surgeons spend their whole career tinkering with the circulation. At the first spike of a temperature I would have taken blood samples for culture. One hand on her cold foot would have warned me of the deterioration hours before it threatened her life. Adrenaline given at progressively higher doses was not the answer. That just helped to switch the kidneys off and once one organ system fails, the rest are likely to follow. At that point I knew she would be dead by the morning. My concerned expression and words of encouragement must have been the last thoughts that poor brain registered in life.

With an air of resignation, I slid down the worn leather armchair in the mansion bar and stared aimlessly at the glass chandelier. I wondered how many young doctors had done the same since World War I and whether they had been as frustrated with life as I was. There had been no news from my other epic weekend cases so my thoughts shifted to the child and his parents at Hemel. I figured Chris would have kept in touch on that score so I called him at home. His wife answered. The man himself had stayed awake most of the night tinkering with the child, but if I really wanted to speak with him she would go and wake him up. I thought for a moment then selfishly said 'yes please.' As it happened, weary Chris was only too happy to share the events of the night with me.

The boy had been quick to regain consciousness after my departure and the drains coming out. Though the nerve blocks reduced the severity of his pain, he was still uncomfortable and fractious. The mother had steadfastly remained by his bedside making every effort to calm him, yet the combination of pain with recall of the fearful accident rendered him hysterical. As a result his drips were avulsed and blood sprayed around the bed.

Chris was not a paediatric anaesthetist by speciality, but having his own children, he could handle the fractious child. Moreover, the wailing and flailing served a useful purpose in the short term. It pushed up his blood

DISAPPOINTMENT

pressure and made the lad breathe deeply and cough just like physiotherapy. That's what he needed at this stage in the proceedings. Chest wall pain and sedation would prevent him from breathing deeply with build-up of carbon dioxide in the blood and narcolepsy.

Once the agitation abated, the exhausted child slept until the early morning. This allowed Chris to insert a new intravenous line then arrange a portable chest X-ray which showed the residual lung to be fully expanded. Beyond the call of duty, Chris even waited for a paediatrician to arrive in the morning to formally hand over After that, as they say, no news from Hemel Hempstead was definitely good news.

It was certainly too late for me to call Ismail in Barnet or Phil at the Central Middlesex so I hoped that the 'no news is good news' adage applied to their patients too. Perhaps I would insist on making post-operative visits tomorrow as an excuse to skip Miss Shepherd's boring outpatient clinic. Then, perhaps I would drive south from Barnet to the Royal Free. Barnet was Mary's own patch so she was intrigued to hear about the case. I was even awarded the phrase 'well done, ruptured aortas are never straightforward.' Perhaps that was an unfortunate reflection on the one that I had assisted her with. About missing outpatients? At first I was subject to that stern, furrowed brow stare, then surprisingly 'I suppose you should show your face. It's the responsible thing to do.' Great, I thought. I've got an afternoon off.

The Central Middlesex and Barnet were in opposite directions. The sensible approach was to phone Phil down in London and gauge whether my appearance was of any interest to him. I asked the switchboard to page him then waited and waited. Perhaps he was scrubbed

THE TRAUMA CHRONICLES

up in theatre. At around 11.30 a.m. I called again and this time he picked up within a couple of minutes.

'Hi Steve, did you bleep me before? I was assisting with a gall bladder.'

I came straight to the point. 'I was planning to swing down and see our patient this afternoon, Phil. Will you be free?' There was a tell-tale pause with an ominous silence. So much so that the embarrassment was palpable ten miles away.

'Oh, sorry Steve. I should have called you. He died yesterday.'

'What did he die from?' I asked indignantly, though I already knew. It had to be heart failure after that crushing blow which burst his pericardial sac.

'His blood pressure just kept drifting down after you left. We kept dialling up the drugs but he went into shock yesterday morning. There was nothing else we could do.'

'There was something you could have done,' I retorted accusingly. 'An intra-aortic balloon pump might have helped. You could have transferred him to the Hammersmith. It's only a mile down the road. I could have arranged that for you.' There was no response. Just loud silence on the end of the phone. I finished with 'make sure he gets an autopsy even if the coroner doesn't insist on one. I have a sense he thrombosed his right coronary artery and I don't want my surgery to be blamed for the death.'

Off I headed across North London towards Barnet on a sunny Tuesday lunch time, eager to surprise my lover at the Royal Free later in the afternoon. Hoping she would be working an early shift and free by 4.30 p.m. A romantic stroll on Hampstead Heath beckoned, or

DISAPPOINTMENT

with luck something more energetic. At Barnet General's reception desk I asked if they could find Ismail for me. If I turned up alone in intensive care no one would know who I was. Conveniently for me he was having lunch in his office and, while I didn't have too much trouble following the directions, office was too generous a term for the cupboard I found him in. One desk, one chair, one window. That was it. There wasn't room enough for two of us to talk there so we wandered up to the nurse's sitting room in the operating theatres. There, he generously introduced me to an uninterested audience of three as the heroic heart and brain surgeon who saved the polytrauma patient over the weekend. As underwhelmed as they were, those words were at least testament to the fact that the man was still alive.

'How's he doing,' I enquired cautiously.

'Not bad,' Ismail said. 'Fine from the cardiovascular standpoint. The chest X-ray looks great and he's breathing on his own. We were waiting for him to wake up before fixing his spine and pelvis. There are some positive signs but he hasn't moved his legs yet.'

'What positive signs?' I enquired with a distinctive hint of disappointment in my voice.

'Well, last night his blood pressure went up and they thought he was coming round. Unfortunately the ITU sedated him again and there's been no response since. I'm still optimistic though.'

'Let's go along and take a look then' I murmured, finishing off a really lousy cup of coffee.

The broken body with a bandaged head lay motionless in a corner of the unit while the breathing machine huffed and puffed noisily. The unusual sound in itself suggested that something had to be wrong with the ventilation. So, first things first, I asked for a stethoscope and could not hear air entering the left lung, the side of the aortic repair. What's more there was a loud squeak as the bellows forced air into the right chest. The computer between my ears was processing these findings when I glanced down at the chest drains which had remained in place since the operation. There were clamps occluding both of them which immediately broadcast the problem. I removed one, and air under tension hissed out through the water in the drainage bottle. Like a huge fart in the bath.

I rounded on the nurse looking after him and growled accusingly.

'Why did you clamp the bloody drains?' She coloured up in panic with a blank stare and I felt reticent about my aggressive tone. Nurses took orders, they didn't make the decisions. Ismail came to her rescue.

'I'm sorry. We routinely clamp chest drains for an hour before removing them. The bleeding stopped a long time ago and I thought you would want us to get them out.'

My response was direct but as polite as I could manage under the circumstances.

'There must be an air leak somewhere from the lung. That was a tension pneumothorax. A few minutes more and he would have arrested.' I'd said enough. The tubes were still bubbling so I was correct about that. It would stop eventually but the drains had to stay in place until it did. Seemingly trivial details meant the difference between life and death in this business. And there's no return ticket once that happens.

I listened again with the stethoscope and the breath sounds had normalised. So had the sounds of the

DISAPPOINTMENT

ventilator. It wasn't straining against resistance any more. Question.

'When was the last chest X-ray?'

'Yesterday in the afternoon,' Ismail replied.

'Let's get one now then, please,' I asked. That meant that I would have to stay in Barnet General for at least another hour waiting to see it. What else could I do? I was visibly pissed off.

It was then that an intensive care doctor sauntered across to say hello. For a second she looked familiar. There followed the inevitable dialogue professing how lucky they had been that I had been available for them at the weekend. Then how extraordinary it had been to operate on a transected aorta and a traumatic cerebral bleed at the same sitting.

'What a clever chap you must be,' she said. Ismail was nodding in agreement and I was getting pumped up by it all. 'I don't know whether you remember me but I was working at the Brompton when you were there,' she continued, 'I was a registrar in chest medicine. We asked you to see a patient once and you came wearing Lord Brock's theatre boots. There was a rumour in the mess that you urinated into them during a long operation—through rubber tubing,' she explained to Ismail. 'We all thought it was hilarious.' She must be posh to use the word urinate, I thought to myself. No one urinates in Scunthorpe.

She was right, of course. It was Christmas and the residents had had a few beers. We'd been caught out late in the evening with a ruptured aorta flown in from Iceland and I'd wondered how I could stand there assisting my irascible German boss for hours on end. Ingenuity saw me through while the tanked up senior registrar made a fool of himself.

101

THE TRAUMA CHRONICLES

'I see you stayed with chest surgery,' she continued. 'You seem well suited to it.'

I didn't know whether that was an insult or a compliment. Those rugby days of my youth were somewhat of a blur. So much so that I wondered if I'd rogered her after a party and didn't recall the experience. So I tried to be discreet.

'Oh yes, of course I remember,' which I didn't. 'I'm doing the stint at Harefield, but soon I'm off to the States to concentrate on cardiac surgery. But I enjoy trauma. It's always a challenge, particularly the peripatetic operating. It's like fighting on a different battlefield every time.'

In retrospect I wondered whether that was the right thing to say. Likening those district general hospitals to a war zone was impolite, but that's how it felt for the last few days. And clearly my mortality rate was going to be substantial.

'I'm Celia. Can I get you both a cup of tea?' Ismail had to get on with an outpatient clinic and, since I was hamstrung until the portable X-ray was taken, that was a welcome suggestion. An opportunity to reminisce about the famous hospital on the Fulham Road that launched my surgical career. But before long I learned her real motive for engaging with me. It surfaced with the line 'while you're here I wonder if you wouldn't mind taking a look at another case for me?' And with that, my 'afternoon off' evaporated.

The patient was in the high dependency part of the unit and not on a ventilator. That said, the little old lady with blue lips was propped bolt upright on her bed, open mouthed and gasping for air. Without asking, two possible diagnoses sprang to mind. The first was chronic

102

DISAPPOINTMENT

bronchitis with emphysema, the common consequence of lifelong smoking. My second guess was lung cancer with compression of the windpipe by tumour spread. Early in my career I had already invented a device to relieve obstruction in such cases, and was frequently asked to do so. The Westaby Tube, it was called, manufactured in Boston, Massachusetts. Not the most famous of my tubes, I might add!

Celia mounted the lady's chest X-ray on the light box and we stood scrutinising it together. The right side with the larger lung was virtually opaque. It was what we call a pleural effusion, yet first attempts to aspirate it through a needle, then evacuate it with a chest drain, had both failed. The poor woman did indeed have emphysema, as was all too obvious in the left lung, but she had also suffered a severe bout of pneumonia. The collection of fluid around the right lung had become infected causing what we term an empyema. Pus solidifies and encases the spongy lung tissue so it no longer expands. Now the combination had tipped her into life-threatening respiratory failure. They had managed to wean her from the breathing machine after a course of antibiotics, but now she was struggling desperately.

Celia spoke to me directly.

'When I heard you were coming back I hoped to persuade you to operate on the old biddy. There's no point just putting her back on the ventilator. We would never get her off it again. If you got her through she's got a very supportive family to look after her. And they've all stopped smoking.'

At that point, the trauma patient's nurse brought us that chest X-ray to review. It looked fine but I already

THE TRAUMA CHRONICLES

had a sinking feeling. There would be no walk on Hampstead Heath at this rate, but what could I do? What I said was 'certainly I'd be pleased to help, but I don't expect they'd be any chance of getting access to an operating theatre or an anaesthetist at short notice. And,' I lied, 'they are expecting me back on call in Harefield this evening.'

'Actually I'd thought of all that' said Celia. 'I'd enquired about it before you arrived, and kept her nil by mouth in case.' She grinned at me sheepishly. My fate was sealed and the best approach was to be gracious about it. I strolled back to the struggling lady's beside, took her cold sweaty hand and said 'Hello luv' in typical northern brogue. 'I'm a surgeon from Harefield Hospital. I've come to make you more comfortable. It means an operation on your chest I'm afraid. Are you OK with that?' She nodded in an enthusiastic way that showed she was too breathless to speak. After a couple of agonisingly heaving breaths she blurted out 'do you think I'll get through?' I didn't honestly know, but what I said was 'of course you will, then I'll want you to buy me a drink afterwards.' That resonated with her and, though gasping for air, she became less tense. The sooner she was asleep the better.

It was 8.30 p.m. when I closed her fragile chest and retired to the theatre rest room. I only had one thought by then. If Sarah was working a late shift she would still be in the hospital. It took a while for someone to pick up the phone on the nurses' station and I was eager to hear her voice. What I heard was 'accident department. Alice speaking, can I help you?'

'I wondered whether Sister McDougall was still on duty?' There followed a brusque 'No, she was working

DISAPPOINTMENT

an early today. On the rota she's doing a late tomorrow.' With that the call was cut off.

With trepidation my next move was to call her shared flat in the nurse's home. Trepidation because I didn't know what response I would generate if I said 'I'm on my way over to see you.'

Barnet was no more than fifteen minutes from the Royal Free and I was iron filings to Sarah's magnet, notwithstanding it should have been five hours earlier. One of her flat mates I recognised answered the phone. I had the distinct impression that she didn't like me very much, and I could imagine her grinning from ear to ear while letting me know that Sarah had gone out for the evening.

Did she know where? Or dare I ask with whom?

'A man' she said pointedly.

So, wearily, I set off back to Harefield with my tail between my legs. When I checked in with the switchboard there was another cheerful message waiting for me.

'Your patient from Wycombe has died.'

Culture Shock

Challenges are what make life interesting and
overcoming them is what makes life meaningful.

Joshua J. Marine

New Year's Eve, 1980, 10.50 a.m. I took off from
Heathrow leaving behind everyone I cared for. There
was little choice in the matter. I was pursuing a fantastic
opportunity that I hoped would define my surgical career.
Late in the afternoon, I stepped down onto the tarmac
at Birmingham Airport. Not Birmingham in England
that shivered in the depths of winter, but Birmingham,
Alabama in America's steamy deep south.

How much did I know about this city that I had
committed to living and working in? The only thing that
mattered was that it housed the world's top academic
cardiac surgery centre. John Kirklin, the man who first
made a success of the heart-lung machine and launched
the specialty in the 1950s, relocated there from the Mayo
Clinic some years before. That's what brought me to the
city now with just a battered suitcase of old clothes to
my name. Aside from the famous medical centre, it was
an industrial steel town like my childhood home. So
after years in London and Cambridge, it was like going
back to my roots.

Thanks to news coverage during my impressionable
teenage years, I knew more about Birmingham than

107

most American cities. This was notorious as America's most racially segregated place. A bastion for white supremacists and flash point for the civil rights activists to rail against blatant discrimination in the Confederacy. Martin Luther King had been arrested there after a violent demonstration. While in prison, he wrote his celebrated 'Letter from Birmingham Jail' addressed to local white ministers in an effort to justify not calling off the march where relentless violence and bloodshed were dealt out by the police. The celebrated epistle was leaked and published widely, together with shocking images of brutality against the demonstrators. Alabama Governor, George Wallace, stood firmly in favour of segregation and was supported by the most aggressive chapters of the Ku Klux Klan. Explosive devices detonated in black homes and churches were so common that the city gained the nickname 'Bombingham, Alabama.'

One notorious event I recall learning about at grammar school. It happened in 1963 after the US Federal Court had ordered the racial integration of Alabama's own state school system. The 16th Street Baptist Church in Birmingham was a meeting place for civil rights activists including Luther King. Children were attending their Sunday School class while many African-American parishioners were gathering outside in the sunshine for their service. Then a bomb detonated, showering the congregation with glass and bricks. Most adults were evacuated but the building collapsed and filled with smoke. Around twenty injured were taken to hospital but, in the grim aftermath, four young black girls were found dead under rubble in the basement.

This was the third bombing by the Ku Klux Klan in two weeks yet, when thousands of angry relatives

CULTURE SHOCK

gathered at the scene, Wallace sent in the state troopers. Extreme violence spread throughout Birmingham and two more demonstrators were shot dead before the US Government sent in the National Guard. Ultimately, the loss of life garnered support for the landmark Civil Rights Act 1964.

From Birmingham Airport, I was heading downtown towards the medical centre, then the Hilton Hotel across the street which would be my home for the first few days. The taxi driver was a talkative chap who seemed to enjoy my English accent, so I asked whether he had been part of those civil rights demonstrations himself. It happened that he was there with the parents of one of the murdered children. Appreciating my interest in the matter, he diverted to 16th street to show me the church itself, rebuilt as a memorial.

It was obvious to me that segregation persisted, if not officially, in practice. I was advised to rent an apartment well away from vexatious downtown in the white suburb of Homewood. Then a new friend gave me a revolver to keep in the glove compartment of my beat up Toyota Corolla because I would be driving to the medical centre in the dark. While that added to the romance of it all, I spent many happy hours in the jazz cellars and speakeasys on the wrong side of the tracks. They seemed to like the English in the deep south. And unsurprisingly, 'Bombingham' was a great place for someone with an interest in trauma surgery.

It was tough going in Dr Kirklin's department. I joined intensive care rounds at 05.00 a.m., scrubbed up in the operating theatres by 07.00 a.m., then toiled in the research laboratory in the evenings. With my degree in biochemistry, I was given a project to investigate the chemical mechanism through which the interaction of blood with foreign surfaces in the heart-lung machine caused a sometimes lethal inflammatory response in the patient. That involved incubating the synthetic materials with human blood in a test tube, then searching for inflammatory triggers generated by the interaction. It was important work that led to a huge discovery when I found those same agents in Kirklin's heart surgery patients. In fact, the concentration of the inflammatory markers in the blood stream at the end of an operation closely correlated with the likelihood of lung or kidney damage. Yet, unsurprisingly, my efforts as a lab rat were often interminably boring. More often than not, I left a technician to process the blood samples while I skipped off to the Emergency room reception area to see which nurses were on duty and join in the action.

It was immediately obvious to me that the levels of care provided for the injured far exceeded those back home. Kirklin was Chief of Staff for surgery overall, not just cardiothoracic surgery, and it seemed to me that all of his departments had limitless resources. Against the backdrop of heavy industry and racial violence in the city, the trauma service was an important specialty in itself. The Americans had learned a considerable amount from the Korean and Vietnam wars where their military surgeons gained massive surgical experience. Helicopters manned by army medics were a necessity in Asia, but had already emerged as the preferred option for transport of trauma patients over long distances in most US states. As early as 1973, the Nationwide Emergency Medical Services Systems Act had established civilian helicopter retrieval programmes together with the

CULTURE SHOCK

training of emergency medical technicians throughout the whole of the United States. I was greatly impressed by the difference that made. Time was of the essence in trauma.

What was the difference between an American trauma centre and an NHS casualty department back in 1981? One might just ask whether a patient bleeding to death from multiple injuries should be treated by a junior hospital doctor diverted from dealing with an asthmatic attack, or a battle-hardened trauma surgeon back from the Vietnam War. Trauma was the leading cause of death across all age groups in England, with over 16,000 patients dying each year. Could the NHS approach be regarded as acceptable? How many patients could be saved by a better system?

While browsing a bookshelf in the Emergency Department, I came across a manual entitled 'Optimal Hospital Resources for the Injured Patient' published back in 1976. It was a detailed document that defined everything necessary in terms of personnel and equipment required for both the pre-hospital setting and Emergency room. What's more, it worked. In the five years since publication, the introduction of specialised trauma facilities had reduced mortality in the seriously injured by 25%. And it definitely made sense to have a trauma centre in an industrial city beset by racial tension and gun culture.

I was sucking an ice cream at the reception desk one steamy summer's night when the red phone rang on the wall. A few well-chosen words put the whole team on alert.

'Incoming to the helipad in ten minutes. Multiple gunshot wounds to the head and chest. In shock.'

In minutes, the duty residents for cardiothoracic and neurosurgery arrived in advance of the patient. Contrast that with my own experience, when I was called to a distant general hospital where the critically injured languished for hours before I could reach them.

There was an established policy in the US to withhold fluid transfusion during helicopter retrieval of patients with penetrating wounds. From experience in warfare the rationale was clear. Those who do not exsanguinate rapidly reach a delicate equilibrium whereby the fall in blood pressure alongside the body's own blood clotting mechanisms conspire to stem life-threatening haemorrhage. To push in clear fluids through a drip with the mistaken objective of normalising blood pressure simply destroys that equilibrium. So much so that a published academic study from Washington DC showed that patients with penetrating wounds had a better chance of survival when brought to hospital by private car rather than the city's advanced life support vehicles. Sad but true.

That very issue emerged as highly controversial in Britain, years later, when pre-hospital resuscitation protocols were advocated under the auspices of the 'Advanced Trauma Life Support' initiative. The guidelines recommended transfusion of substantial volumes of intravenous fluid in the pre-hospital setting for patients with so called low blood pressure, where 'low' was interpreted as less than 100 mm Hg. But from a cardiac surgeon's perspective, that pressure is very far from life-threatening.

I addressed the pre-hospital resuscitation debate later in my career when I started writing textbooks on the subject. In *Cardiothoracic Trauma*, published in 1999,

CULTURE SHOCK

leading Houston trauma surgeon Ken Mattox wrote this on the subject:

For victims of penetrating thoracic trauma the administration of pre-hospital resuscitation fluids has a detrimental effect when compared with delaying fluid resuscitation until skin incision. These data also appear to be true for blunt chest injury.

Time in the Emergency room should not be used as an opportunity to 'volume load' a patient who has chest trauma. Such aggressive fluid administration results in increased lung water and consolidation. If anything this is a time to consciously restrict clear fluid volume loading because of the numerous complications associated with aggressive fluid resuscitation.

This was an opinion formulated through years of experience in the military and on the front line of civilian trauma care in a well organised system. Compare that with my experience over that long weekend's operating, when the patients were awash with cold clear fluid and their blood wouldn't clot. Ultimately the buck stops with the surgeon so it is discouraging to start on the back foot when protocol-driven resuscitation efforts have rendered a daunting task virtually impossible.

The next revelation late that evening was that the radiographers who operated the whole body CT scanner were preparing to receive the patient. CT stands for computed tomography. The technique emerged through innovative developments in both X-ray and computer science and provided images of the body in cross sections. The method was developed by EMI scientists in Britain and revolutionised diagnosis within the brain and body cavities in the early 1970s.

Though the first CT scanner was installed at Northwick Park Hospital in north London in 1975, the NHS was slow to commission others. Needless to say the Mayo Clinic and Massachusetts General Hospital soon introduced the machines to the United States and, by the time the inventor received his Nobel Prize in 1978, more than 200 had been installed in American hospitals. I worked for years in major teaching hospitals in London and Cambridge, and still hadn't seen one. It was a money thing, but for trauma and cancer patients it made a huge difference to the speed of diagnosis and timing of surgery.

Like an excited schoolboy, I went up onto the roof to watch the helicopter land. I guess that was the crux of my time in America. Being part of something that seemed light years ahead of the situation back home. In Alabama, civilian gunshot wounds transported by air was simply a continuation of their Vietnam War experience. The message was straightforward. Get life-threatening injuries to the surgeon as quickly as possible. Don't tinker around by the roadside or in the street. The operating theatre is the place to fix people. It was then and it is now.

This patient was full of holes. Four bullet wounds to the trunk and one to the head but he was still breathing spontaneously and had a measurable blood pressure. The fact that he was alive told us that the bullets had missed the major arteries in the chest and those in the brain stem that kept him breathing. Strapped securely to the trolley, he was downloaded from the helicopter, groaning loudly with each bump along the way. A lift from the helipad

CULTURE SHOCK

brought him directly down into the Emergency room where the trauma team were waiting. The whole process worked like clockwork. The anaesthetist inserted a large bore cannula into a vein in the left arm while nurses and Emergency room technicians in aprons and rubber gloves cut away the blood-soaked clothing. He was African-American, making it impossible to gauge the blood loss from skin pallor, but he was sweaty and cold with a rapid pulse that was barely palpable at the wrist.

Judging from the entry wounds apparent when he was rolled to remove the bloodied shirt, he had been shot in the back from close range with low velocity bullets. Another had passed through his skull entering above the right ear and blowing out an exit wound high in the forehead. This suggested, even to me, that he was attempting to escape from an assailant who was determined to kill him. Was that the police, I wondered? Not that it mattered. The routine didn't differ between saints or sinners.

That first cannula was used to render him unconscious from his agitated state and to prevent interference with the resuscitation efforts. Needless to say, the anaesthetic further compromised his blood pressure. As the slug of barbiturate left the syringe the readings were announced loudly to all present.

'I get 70/40 in the right arm.'

'That's fine,' responded the anaesthetist. 'Put in another IV and I'll do the neck line when I've intubated him.'

That meant working around those holes in his head hidden by matted hair and slimy blood clot. Pulling back on his square chin, the curved metal plate of the laryngoscope slid deftly over a purple tongue, past his fleshy tonsils and into the cartilaginous entrance of the voice box. Straight ahead were the twitching vocal cords waiting for the stiff tracheal tube to be thrust between them. Performed expertly, the plastic tube with its inflatable cuff secures the airway and the means to push oxygen into the lungs. Hopefully.

In this case, frothy blood foamed up the lumen from the shattered right lung. A stethoscope confirmed air entry into the left lung but no breath sounds at all on the right. Only after evacuating blood and air with a drain could the peppered right lung re-expand. The vital signs were called out again.

'Blood pressure now 60/35, heart rate 118.'

'Ok, squeeze in some O negative blood through the warmer,' came the considered response from the team leader. 'Hold off on the clear fluid for now. Just ease the pressure back up to 80 again. No higher for now.'

The response to one bag of blood was encouraging. It nudged up the pressure appropriately, suggesting that there was no cardiac tamponade. One might imagine that any gunshot wound involving the heart would prove rapidly fatal, but that is not necessarily the case even in my own experience. I recall one young man where a handgun bullet passed straight through his heart and lodged in the opposite chest wall. The equilibrium of cardiac tamponade saved him because he had no prehospital fluids. After I sewed up both ends he did fine.

I sensed that the junior resident delegated to insert the chest drain was inexperienced and nervous. More directly, he was faffing around. He was asking for local anaesthetic when the guy was already unconscious and was unsure about where to site the tube. 'Let me give you a hand with that' I offered politely, and he was happy

CULTURE SHOCK

to accept. In seconds, I'd shoved the scalpel followed by the drain on its introducer deeply into the chest cavity, aiming it away from the heart. As the introducer was withdrawn, blood and air pissed out to fill the drainage bottle and the breath sounds became audible again. Bingo. A lifesaving intervention in two minutes. 'I see you've done that before,' remarked the anaesthetist, who didn't know me from Adam.

There were soon signs of improvement, but blood and bubbles continued to drain from the chest tube. And one pressing issue needed to be resolved. With bullet wounds to both head and chest, which needed surgery first? Besides the blood there were grey fragments of brain in his hair. Moreover, the pupil of the left eye was more dilated than the right suggesting an element of brain compression. That said, it still constricted when a torch was shone into the eyes, a positive sign that confirmed the all-important brain stem was intact.

With a degree of stability it was time to define his injuries, not just with the plain x-rays that I was used to, but with that fancy contraption the CT scanner. Images in three dimensions. Pictures created in just a few minutes would show the precise path of the bullets, the injuries they inflicted and where they came to rest. The surgeons could then plan their approach with defined aims in mind. This was not the speculative opening of Pandora's box that I was forced to adopt at home. The scanner would reveal the damage and show what needed to be done to retrieve the situation.

As the dark blue trickle of blood continued to fill the drainage bottle his blood pressure was drifting down again. Consequently, the decision to operate first on the

THE TRAUMA CHRONICLES

chest was inevitable even before the CT scans appeared. Scans wouldn't change the fact that persistent bleeding had declared itself the priority. So the patient and chest surgeons were on their way to the operating theatre even before the pictures were ready.

Given the invitation to scrub in, I took the first assistant's place while the resident mounted the pictures on the X-ray viewing box. It was the first time I had seen CT scans which proved a revelation to me. Much of the blood and air had been evacuated by the drain allowing the lung to re-expand. Blood filled tracks were visible where the low velocity bullets had passed through the tissues and ricocheted around the pleural cavity. Two were clearly visible. One had fragmented after splintering a rib and running out of steam. Another lay spent on the diaphragm. Mysteriously, there was another entry wound in his back where the shoulder blade had been shattered, yet there was no sign of a third bullet on the head, neck and chest scans. Nor was there an exit wound to explain it. Very strange. Ominous in fact.

Opening the chest between ribs is like prising open a clam. It's like lifting the bonnet of a car to find what's wrong with the engine. In this case, liquid blood sploshed loudly into the sucker, then purple clot slithered out silently like a snake before slopping onto the floor. We asked our anaesthetist to deliberately block air from entering the right lung so the airless lobes would deflate to a fraction of their size, making it easier to inspect the chest wall for bleeding. As anticipated, there seemed to be no damage to the heart or main arteries, but there was obvious bleeding from the root of the lung. A bullet had entered the lower of the two large veins which carry blood back from the lung into the left side of the heart.

CULTURE SHOCK

Given that it was a low pressure vessel, the rate of blood loss was limited. Moreover, it was simple to fix with a couple of well-placed stitches and, thankfully, most of the bleeding from the penetrated lung tissue itself had stopped spontaneously. That was the benefit of preserving his own clotting system.

As we fished out the two spent bullets it dawned on me what may have happened to the third. The vanishing missile had moved on. 'Bullet embolus' was something I first encountered in Harlem, New York City, during my scholarship years before. Having entered a blood vessel, the flow pushes the missile onwards. In this case from the lung's vein into the collecting chamber, known as the left atrium. From there it had simply rolled on through the mitral valve, appropriately named after a bishop's mitre, then into the main pumping chamber, the left ventricle. This powerful muscle is capable of shooting a foreign body out through the aortic valve and round the arterial system. Many missiles are too large to enter the vessels to the brain and cause stroke. They tend to be pushed on through the circulation until they obstruct an artery to the leg. Sure enough when the issue was raised, we found his right leg was colder than the left and no pulses could be felt in it. That was the only bullet embolus of my career and, ultimately, it was a simple procedure to extract it through a small incision in the groin.

Locating that last bullet was important, but not as crucial as decompressing the pulped and swollen brain. The chest wounds were unlikely to kill him now. A gunshot wound to the head quite possibly would. Given the site of the entry and exit wounds, the bullet would have passed through a couple of lobes of the brain above eye level but it had not crossed the midline. More importantly, the trajectory kept it away from the brain stem and critical blood vessels. The cheerful neurosurgery resident chipped in that 90% of these patients die before reaching hospital, while half of those who arrive succumb before leaving the Emergency room. Once again, this man was a self-selected survivor given appropriate treatment.

It was extraordinary to view a CT scan of the head for the first time. It was almost like having a life sized model of the brain with all its lobes and convolutions then the trauma drawn onto it. On the screen was an oval section through the head surrounded by shattered bright white skull bone containing grey brain matter inside. Through that passed a fluffy line like the vapour trail from an aeroplane, the path of the hand gun bullet from the site it smashed its way into the head to the place it managed to exit. Under the entry point, bright spicules of bone had entered the grey brain matter. Where it departed, larger bone fragments lay beneath the scalp like a sunburst. Fascinating how aesthetic a buggered brain can be.

The so called 'vapour trail in the stratosphere' was blood clot within cavitated nervous tissue, then beneath the exit wound was a collection of blood that markedly distorted the brain's anatomy. This 'subdural haematoma' accounted for the unequal pupils. Old fashioned skull x-rays would reveal only parts of this pathology so seeing the damage in a computerised reconstruction was a complete revelation.

For me the brain was like a lump of jelly in a ceramic dish. You don't cut it or stitch it as in other types of surgery. It's a matter of drilling windows through the

CULTURE SHOCK

bone then carefully sucking out fragments of grey or white brain matter with the consistency of blancmange. Or, in this case, shattered strawberry 'Jell-O' as the Americans called it. Besides the blood clot, there was enough swelling on the scan to mandate a brain decompression procedure. That involved drilling a series of strategically situated burr holes and cutting through the bone between them with an oscillating saw then lifting it away to relieve pressure. The detached piece of skull would be kept clean in a fridge then replaced beneath the scalp when the swelling abated. As long as the man survived, that is. The fact that he was semi-conscious and breathing spontaneously on admission were good prognostic signs; the resuscitation had been prompt and measured so as not to increase pressure inside the skull. A bullet that destroys the right hemisphere of the brain might leave the patient with restricted movement or sensation of the left half of the body, but other brain functions including cognition, memory, speech and vision are controlled by both hemispheres. They should remain intact if the decompression proved effective.

Brain surgeons tend to be different personality types from heart surgeons. I used to describe us—the thoracics— as the special forces and them as the Intelligence Corps. I was keen to see what a gunshot wound to the brain actually looked like up close so I stayed in the operating room until the early hours to watch. The procedure was a bit like taking the top off a lightly boiled egg and having the yolk spill out. Except this yolk was red and the shattered brain like rice pudding. Sucker not scalpel territory. It was a matter of gently extracting detached grey matter while preserving everything that remained.

Strange to contemplate what thoughts passed through that mush before the missile struck.

When the debridement was complete the surface of the brain was washed with saline solution and every last bleeder cauterised before stitching closed the scalp. Very different from the cut and thrust of chest surgery I was used to.

There was no time to head back to Homewood only to turn round and come back again. I spent an hour or so in the back seat of my car, then showered in the surgeons' changing room, and started all over again with a change of theatre blues. It was a sequence I would repeat many times in my career. Sleep was a waste of time with such a wealth of exciting experience there to be learned.

Downtime gave me the chance to think about other things. What remained of the wreck of my personal life. I pictured my daughter Gemma in Cambridge tucking into breakfast. Then I wondered what Sarah was doing at that precise time. I figured it would be 10 in the morning. Maybe she was on an early shift in the accident department or just leaving after a long night. The alternatives I didn't care to consider. It was me who had chosen to leave and I couldn't lock her away in a convent. I recalled her animated description of that murdered patient with a gunshot wound to the head. How some insisted that it wasn't worth trying to resuscitate him. Ultimately they were correct but it wasn't going to deter her from trying. I wondered whether she ever thought about me in her busy London life or had she moved on? Another doctor perhaps, or a wealthy banker. The world was her oyster and I needed to stop ruminating about the fact. So I went off to the operating theatre to start another Alabama day.

CULTURE SHOCK

What was so different about Birmingham? What would be the likelihood of urgent chest then brain operations within an hour of arriving at a hospital in London? Nil in my experience, and that brought a disturbing analogy to mind. It was the difference between the super fit, well drilled University of Alabama American footballers working through their playbook, versus the rag, tag and bobtail efforts of my medical school rugby team after a hard night on the beer. Alabama's 'Crimson Tide' were top of the National College Football league and I would watch their cheerleaders' practice routines in a gym close to the medical centre. Amateur night really doesn't cut it when it comes to saving lives and I guess that summed up the attitude I brought back to London when I returned to complete my so-called training.

Then came the watershed moment for my whole career. It was 05.30 on Friday 24 July, 1981. As I arrived for the intensive care round there was a palpable buzz of excitement amongst the residents around the first patient's bed despite the fact that he was dying. Naturally I was curious. It happened that the previous evening at the Texas Heart Institute, Dr Denton Cooley had implanted the world's second total artificial heart. This was a full 14 years after the disastrous first, given the huge controversy the operation generated between rival research groups. Nonetheless I was determined to see it so that evening I took the red eye flight to Houston.

In the early hours before sunrise I boarded a night bus from the airport, drifted past the glittering skyline and on to the sprawling medical centre. Having finally found the Texas Heart Institute, I pushed a couple of chairs together in the reception area and fell asleep. At 06.00 that Saturday morning a receptionist arrived and politely enquired as to whether she could assist me with anything. I'm sure she suspected that I was a tramp and I looked and smelled that way. Undeterred I proudly announced in my best English accent that I was a heart surgeon from London and had come to meet Dr Cooley and see his artificial heart patient. I also mentioned that the great man and I had both trained at the Brompton Hospital in London, so I was sure he would be pleased to receive me.

'That's a coincidence,' she replied. Dr Cooley has just walked in the entrance behind you.'

And so it was that the interloper from Scunthorpe met the world's most famous cardiac surgeon. Tall, handsome and imposing just as heart surgeons should be. More to the point he was polite and understanding particularly when I told him that I was working with the revered Dr Kirklin and we had both been residents under the mitral valvotomy pioneer Oswald Tubbs on the Fulham Road. That seemed like a million miles away now.

Dr Cooley treated me with great kindness. Despite it being the weekend his secretary arrived at 06.30 and made us tea. I was then given a tour of the intensive care unit with one hundred beds, the operating suite with twenty-four rooms and then to his museum for a photograph with the great man. I was like a dog with two tails but by the afternoon the patient was not doing well. Not only was the bulky pulsating device destroying the red blood cells it was compressing and obstructing the veins from the lungs causing what we call pulmonary oedema. Another new technique, extracorporeal membrane oxygenation, was being used to treat low blood oxygen levels and support the circulation until a

CULTURE SHOCK

donor heart could be found. Needless to say Dr Cooley was disappointed, but he still found time to call one of his attractive perfusionists and request that she show me Houston on a Saturday night—but that promising liaison didn't last long. The transplant happened overnight, the girl was called in and I had my first sight of a total artificial heart within the chest. I was hooked of course and could have flown back to Birmingham without the plane. Sadly, the outcome was the same as for the first attempt. The donor heart failed and the man died within a week. Nevertheless, within weeks new artificial heart programmes had emerged in the US, Russia, China, Japan and in several European countries, Britain excluded. Coincident with this disappointment, the artificial heart engineer Robert Jarvik of Utah wrote in *Scientific American*, 'If the artificial heart is ever going to achieve its objectives it must be more than a pump, more than functional, reliable and dependable. It must be forgettable.' By that he meant that implanted blood pumps should not impact negatively upon the patient's quality of life. High ambition, but one I would pursue throughout my practice. Indeed I had a career-long association with the Texas Heart Institute and ultimately received the highest honour from them for my efforts. One that Dr Kirklin himself had received.

Alabama in the Autumn is magical. The Fall they call it over there. The nights were still balmy and many of the nurse anaesthetists and surgical technicians lived close by. We would hang out by the pool drinking until midnight then back into the hospital at 05.00 for the morning rounds. Late that October I spoke at a conference in Chattanooga, then was driven back to Birmingham by some of the residents. They wanted

125

to show me their glorious countryside before it was too late. So we drifted south by Lookout Mountain, meandering through canyons and splendid rock formations. I sat enthralled by mile upon mile of bright yellow poplars, scarlet dogwoods, orange maples and golden hickories now shedding their leaves to provide a spectacular warm carpet beneath. Simple wonders of nature that were worth saving lives for, and I wondered to myself, 'Am I really going back to London and leave all of this?'

Then something else magical happened. Sarah came. This wasn't her first trip to the States, she had a cousin she'd visited in Washington. But this trip wasn't a vacation. It had a compelling purpose for her. Though she never verbalised it I could tell that she had critical decisions to make in her life. So when I tried to embrace her at the airport gate she backed away, froze and avoided physical contact. Not even a kiss. Her body language made it known that she was angry with me, and I sensed she must be close to someone else. This was an expedition to shake things down. What did the flash, philandering surgeon in America really mean to her? She had already lost one home and secure future through my relentless pursuit but then I disappeared. Buggered off in the depths of the London winter. Leaving her with just a suitcase full of clothes and my photograph in that dismal hospital tower block in Hampstead. Worse still she knew me all too well. She understood that I would be spinning around in an ivory tower of an American heart hospital. 'Flash Harry' surrounded by amorous nurses keen to entertain the cad with the posh English accent. I'd long lost the Scunthorpe dialect by then, not that it mattered in the steamy deep South.

CULTURE SHOCK

It was an hour's drive from the airport to my apartment. First through downtown and the industrial heartland, then past the sprawling medical centre and finally over the 'mountain' to the Confederate enclave of Homewood.

'It's very different from the North,' she murmured quietly, staring away from me through the dusty windscreen. 'Do you have a girlfriend here?' she asked, as if concerned about what she might discover. I said 'no.' That approximated to the truth. I was an opportunist who took what came his way. Polyamorous some people call it these days, but I couldn't visualise a woman like Sarah staying celibate either. She looked stunning as always though I thought she had lost weight. For once something other than cardiac surgery occupied my frontal lobes, though sadly not my private parts. So we sat and chatted under the stars, suitably sedated by Californian chardonnay.

Next day was Halloween and I'd been invited to watch Auburn play Louisiana State University down south in Montgomery. I loved American football, the crunch of shoulders, crash of helmets and brute force of it all. We set off together as the sun came up and this time the dialogue, like the weather, was warmer. Perhaps for the first time ever we were actually doing something together. Then after the game I just kept on driving. I wanted to share the glorious Alabama countryside in the Fall with her. That would make her journey memorable if nothing else, so we drifted through Oak Mountain State Park then down the I-65 highway towards Mobile. Endless avenues of amber and crimson under the bright blue sky. I knew what I was doing, needless to say. The psychologist in me was determined to draw her in again so I was heading for Florida, then turn left. There was the spectacular Gulf Coast.

I aimed to reach Fort Walton beach before sunset. Mile upon mile of powdery white sand and warm emerald sea which I knew would remind her of the Kenyan coast. Happy times at Malindi where the tomboy in her fished for marlin under the blistering sun with her father. I suspected some guy was eagerly awaiting her Hampstead homecoming so this was my last chance. The sea shore had to be the place to woo her again. Should that prove successful, I needed to treat her with respect this time.

'Where are we going?' Sarah asked.

'I don't know,' I responded, 'but as long as you're with me I don't care.'

Real Charlotte Bronte stuff, though some might say Enid Blyton. What was the more romantic, a blistering deep red sunset over the Gulf of Mexico or a rainy Halloween evening in Belsize Park? What's more I was tanned by deep South sunshine and ripped through gym work outs with the cheerleaders. Of course Sarah had to decide who and what she wanted in her life. I was simply nudging her in my direction. Now was the time for my rape and pillage days to stop if I was to fulfil my destiny as respected surgeon one day. I'd left far too much misery in my wake already, which I deeply regretted.

Later that evening we strolled hand in hand along am empty beach, listening to water lap on the sand and watching the glorious sun sink into the sea.

'Did you ever watch Gone with the Wind?' I asked.

'No I don't believe I did,' she whispered, as if anticipating some profound statement.

'Me neither,' I quipped pathetically. A lie but it made her laugh and broke the ice. It had been a happy day. She was calmer and the anger had abated. Soon it was dark with just fishing boats out on the water and the harbour lights of Destin in the distance. 'We're 250 miles from Homewood,' I said. 'That's a four hour drive at best. Shall we find a hotel?' Sarah nodded in the affirmative. What else could I say but 'one room or two?'

I did succeed in identifying the pathological basis of the 'Post Perfusion Syndrome' together with the foreign materials in the bypass circuit that triggered a lethal 'whole body inflammatory response.' When the manufacturers of the heart-lung machine components removed nylon, cardiac surgery became safer overnight and innumerable lives were saved. Did the importance of that contribution sink in? Not at the time but I was invited to give lectures on the landmark discovery in a number of top American cardiac centres including Johns Hopkins and the Mayo Clinic. Inevitably I was asked whether I would stay in the United States and I was tempted from the professional standpoint. But I couldn't abandon my family.

Washington DC was our last stop before flying back to Heathrow. Sarah would see her cousin again and I would take up a long standing invitation to visit the famous MedStar Trauma Centre.

The American Way

Before you diagnose yourself with depression or
low self-esteem, first make sure you are not just
surrounded by assholes.

Sigmund Freud

During January 1982, the whole of North America
was bitterly cold. Even Birmingham was paralysed by
snow, so much so that Dr Kirklin instructed the surgical
teams to take up residence in the Hilton Hotel across
the street from the medical centre. Having relinquished
the apartment in Homewood, we joined my colleagues
there before finally heading to London. The send-off
was more than I deserved.

Ironically it was Friday the thirteenth when we were
due to fly. First leg, Birmingham to Washington National
Airport but it was uncertain as to whether the plane
could take off. Ice and snow rapidly re-accumulated on
the runway as soon as it was cleared and by then I was
already a week late in beginning my post at the Hospital
for Sick Children. Not a distinguished homecoming with
others having to cover for me.

Could things get worse? They certainly could.
Having set off with a degree of trepidation, we were
in bumpy clouds five miles from touching down when
the landing was aborted. It was 4.05 pm, already dark
and in the midst of a blizzard so the sudden change

THE TRAUMA CHRONICLES

caused considerable unease in the aircraft. We weren't told very much. Simply that there was a problem on the ground and it might be necessary to divert to Baltimore. Given the dire circumstances the announcement was an understatement. Minutes earlier, Air Florida flight 90 that had been destined for Fort Lauderdale crashed into the 14th Street Bridge conveying Interstate 395 over the Potomac River. The aircraft had been airborne for just 30 seconds reaching an altitude of 352 feet before it smashed down on the bridge hitting seven vehicles and demolishing 30 metres of guard rail. Four motorists were killed instantly and four others seriously injured before the shattered fuselage plunged through thick ice and into the freezing water.

An emergency rescue response was mounted at 4.07 pm but in appalling road conditions and rush hour traffic it took the ambulances twenty minutes to reach the bridge. By then, seventy of the seventy-four passengers, and four of five crew members were dead. Clinging to the tail section above the ice was one flight attendant and the other survivors, but with two feet of snow on the riverbank and ice floes in the river, the rescuers were unable to reach them.

At 4.20 pm as we were circling above waiting to land, a US Park Police helicopter bravely hovered low over the ice and attempted to hoist those able to cooperate to the shore. Intrepid passers-by also entered the treacherous river to make dire rescue attempts. Sadly, two of the initial survivors subsequently succumbed. One was unable to extricate himself from tangled wreckage which eventually submerged while the second heroically swam to assist others but drowned before reaching the bank himself.

THE AMERICAN WAY

The disaster was attributed to pilot error. Neither had sufficient experience of flying in winter weather conditions. Initially they encountered difficulty in pushing back from the gate in snow and failed to switch on the engines' ice protection system. It took 49 minutes to taxi to the take-off runway and when heavy lumps of ice accumulated on the wings they fruitlessly relied upon exhaust fumes from a DC9 in front to melt it. There had been a question about whether to abort the take-off but my plane and others were scheduled to land shortly on that same runway.

Just half an hour after the flight 90 incident, the Washington Metro experienced its first fatal train crash at Federal Triangle Station. Thus Washington's nearest airport, the main bridge into the city and one of the busiest subway lines all closed simultaneously, paralysing much of the metropolis. MedStar was busy that evening but we managed to land after an hour's delay. Welcome to Washington.

I first met the affable Howard Champion, Director of MedStar, when I was training in general surgery in Cambridge and listened to him lecture on the Birmingham Accident Hospital Trauma Course. Howard is an Englishman by birth though his father was an Australian surgeon with the 8th Army in North Africa during World War II. When I told him my father had been there too with the RAF he invited me for a couple of beers and a natter at the end of the day. In short, we had much in common and got on like a house on fire.

After beginning his career in Edinburgh, Howard moved to train at the Accident Hospital with Britain's doyen of trauma surgery, Peter London. Greatly impressed by their emergency surgical team rota, he introduced the Birmingham modus operandi to the University of Maryland after emigrating to the US in 1972. The rest is history, as they say. Right place, right time. He was a mover and shaker who wanted to make a difference.

The Director of Trauma in Maryland was the charismatic cardiac surgeon Adams Cowley, whose principal interest was shock. Cowley had served with the US Army in wartime Europe where he recognised that patients with severe wounds could generally be saved if they reached a surgeon and had their bleeding stopped within an hour. He referred to shock as 'a momentary pause in the act of death,' but, once set in motion in those historical times, it was usually irreversible.

On his return to the US, the army awarded Cowley a huge grant to establish a small shock trauma research unit in Baltimore. Though this attracted patients from far and wide, many referred to the four bed unit as the 'death lab,' and from here the 'Golden Hour' principle ultimately emerged. Cowley would emphasise 'if you are critically injured you have less than 60 minutes to reach help. You might not die right then. It may be three days or two weeks later, but within that hour something has happened in your body that is irreparable.' He was right about that. Urgent blood transfusion in the field slowed the deterioration but clear fluids that do not carry oxygen certainly couldn't.

With a continuous stream of trauma patients it was possible for Cowley to identify the complex physiological changes that defined the shock state. Put simply, shock develops after a widespread reduction in tissue blood flow and oxygen delivery. As pressure falls within the circulation during bleeding, receptors in the blood vessel walls cause reflex constriction of the small arteries in an attempt to compensate. The automated component of the nervous system responds by causing rapid heart rate, sweating, pallor and coldness of the skin. Veins also constrict which can lead to difficulty in placing an intravenous cannula. Finally, over-extraction of oxygen from sluggish blood flow causes the blue skin discoloration we call cyanosis.

Cowley established that bleeding of less than 10% of the circulatory volume is well tolerated by fit patients. Compensatory mechanisms simply draw in fluid from the tissues to restore blood volume in less than twenty-four hours. Even loss of 20% of the circulating volume is unlikely to drop the blood pressure significantly. Flow to the brain and heart muscle are selectively preserved by automatic reduction in flow to the gut, liver and other organs. But when blood loss exceeds 30%, flow to skin and muscles shuts down to the extent that oxygen deprivation causes damage to the tissues with acid production. Then agitation and restlessness emerge as early clinical signs. Ultimately, prolonged haemorrhagic shock causes tissue inflammation and permanent injury so that the liver releases toxins and the lungs fill with fluid. Herein there were distinct similarities with the damaging effects of cardiopulmonary bypass. Death will follow if the Golden Hour lapses without treatment so the first objective is to stop the blood loss. Surgeons do that.

It was Cowley who persuaded his military contemporaries to use their helicopters to transport patients into the unit more rapidly, but they had difficulty in convincing the Maryland State Police to allow it. So he cleverly agreed to share the helicopters with them. The first Medevac retrieval happened in 1969 after the opening of Baltimore's five storey, thirty-two bed Academic Centre for the Study of Trauma. It was a revolutionary move for its time since conventional ambulances in Europe and the United States carried limited medical equipment. The drivers would do little more than load up the patient and convey them directly to the nearest hospital, where they would be received by inexperienced junior doctors. As Cowley pointed out, the local hospital was usually ill-equipped with the specialists needed to treat severe injuries.

Cowley and Champion also changed the road transport of trauma victims by introducing emergency medical technicians in well-equipped ambulances to serve the Baltimore region. Inevitably, such reorganisation required political support which only happened after a close friend of Maryland's Governor Mandel was severely injured in a motor accident and brought to the trauma centre. Having survived against the odds the young prosecutor, and subsequent Congressman, Dutch Ruppersberger, asked Cowley how he could repay him. Cowley responded 'you can run for office and help raise the resources we need to continue saving lives.' Ruppersberger did successfully run for local, state and federal office and proceeded to fly the flag for the Baltimore Shock Trauma system. Soon afterwards the 'nearest hospital first' policy was abandoned in the US.

Mandel soon issued an executive order to launch the Maryland Institute for Emergency Medicine with Cowley as director. It was into this facilitatory environment that Champion introduced the Birmingham Accident Hospital trauma team ethos in 1975. It fitted well with

THE AMERICAN WAY

Cowley's plans and, between them, they established the Maryland Shock Trauma Centre as the world's leading institution for the treatment of major injuries. Ironic then that the inspirational Birmingham Accident Hospital went unsupported. The old brick building next to the brewery was closed by the NHS in 1993 without any recognition that its life-saving protocols were used to launch the US system of trauma care.

Before Champion advocated the surgical trauma team policy, the Emergency Department was run by physicians. To implement the controversial changes, he designed a new reception area specifically for major injuries which he named the Medical and Shock Trauma Acute Resuscitation unit, or MedStar. The six purpose-built resuscitation bays with their own radiology unit were linked directly to the helicopter landing pad, ambulance bays and operating theatres at the base of the hospital's intensive care tower. And because the department was now manned by surgeons, it eliminated the delays inherent in accessing immediate surgery for life-threatening injuries.

Champion's next move was to collaborate with the State Police Department to purchase two BK117 helicopters specifically for MedStar, then persuade all three Washington University Hospitals, together with DC General Hospital, to join a collaborative trauma system with MedStar at its heart. It was a highly political move. Some supported the introduction of specialist trauma surgery and intensive care, others viewed it as threatening competition with an inevitable loss in revenue. Ultimately, it was the inordinate frequency of knife and gunshot wounds in the city that persuaded the politicians of the need for a focused approach. So prolific were penetrating injuries that all three divisions of the US Armed Forces medical services taught their trauma modules at the Washington Hospital Center. Indeed, none of their own military hospitals received trauma or emergency patients. And eventually trainees from the British military gravitated there, including the special forces.

There were still battles to be fought on the pre-hospital front. Firstly the District of Columbia ambulance service worked in tandem with the Fire Department, not the hospitals. During the Vietnam War there was a policy to counter bleeding and raise blood pressure using dilute salt or sugar solutions. These clear fluids leaked out of the circulation, so were used in the ratio of 3 litres of clear fluid for every suspected litre of blood lost. In time, the use of so called crystalloid fluids was advocated by the Advanced Trauma Life Support course which taught that two litres of fluid should be rapidly infused into any patient considered at risk of haemorrhagic shock. Unfortunately, the inevitable redistribution into the tissues caused waterlogging of the lungs, gut and even heart muscle, alongside disturbances in blood biochemistry and immune function. That is what Howard had talked about on the Birmingham Accident Hospital course I attended and it resonated with me.

While litres of cold clear fluid might raise the blood pressure of patients with broken bones needing orthopaedic operations, it frustratingly rendered surgery of the internal organs more difficult than it already was. Only red blood cells carry oxygen so both of us considered it conceptually wrong. What's more, the emergency medical technicians were spending far too long trying to insert cannulas in collapsed veins

THE AMERICAN WAY

at the accident site which added further risk to the situation. Howard bitterly described one incident where interminable faffing around trying to obtain venous access had concluded with fatal exsanguination from a jugular vein. All they needed to do was to press on the bleeding site and get to hospital. Anyone could ligate a low pressure vein.

So how did the ubiquitous Advanced Trauma Life Support (ATLS) protocol come about? That's an interesting story that I was told after seeing a poster advertising the course in Alabama. I already knew about the Advanced Cardiac Life Support programme, but its trauma equivalent was a recent addition borne out of personal tragedy.

An orthopaedic surgeon, Dr James Styner of Lincoln, Nebraska, had attended a Valentine's Day party with his family in Los Angeles. On 17 February 1976 he set out for home piloting a twin engine, six seater plane containing his wife and four children. They flew east over Southern California, crossing Arizona before touching down in New Mexico to refuel. Continuing over the southern Rockies and Kansas they had reached Nebraska when they encountered low cloud. Five hours into the flight Styner became disorientated and lost altitude. It was 6pm and already dark. Charlene, his wife, was sitting in the co-pilot's seat but not buckled in. The four children were behind with the youngest, a three-year-old girl, sitting on her brother's knee. Tragically, the plane was far too low. It hit a row of trees at 168 mph ripping off both wings and rupturing the fuel tanks. Could anyone survive that?

A gaping hole was torn along the right side of the aircraft as it dropped into a thicket then rocketed on into

139

a field. It was then that a piece of shattered propeller from the left engine flew through the pilot's window, missed James, but smashed into the side of Charlene's skull. The impact launched her 300 feet outside the fuselage where she died instantly. James remained conscious but with facial lacerations and fractured ribs. Two of the children were rendered deeply unconscious with skull fractures, one of whom was impaled by tangled metal in the wreckage.

Soon after impact, everything fell silent under a full moon as the temperature dipped below freezing. It took time to register the reality of the situation but, with no signs of help in the vicinity, James set about extricating his children from the crumpled wreck. Given an immediate risk of hypothermia he gathered clothing from the scattered suitcases and made a bed within the remains of the plane to keep the unconscious children warm. The first two desperate attempts to find Charlene were fruitless. He finally located her broken body during the third search and thought her to be dead. Yet as human nature dictates, James went back to his wife three more times to be sure nothing could be done. Each time she was colder and ghostly pale in the moonlight as *rigor mortis* set in.

While shivering there in the broken fuselage in the early hours, it became apparent from distant lights that there was a road several hundred yards away. With his children still unconscious, the injured Styner had no choice other than to set out to find help. Eventually he managed to flag down a married couple in a car who succeeded in driving to the crash site. They loaded all the injured passengers into the one vehicle then drove them to a rural hospital several miles away.

THE AMERICAN WAY

What happened next was the stimulus for the Advanced Trauma Life Support course but for all the wrong reasons. The muddy, wet, bloodied band arrived at the emergency reception area to find the door locked. After banging for some time a startled night nurse opened the door but wouldn't allow anyone in until the doctors arrived from home. These were two general practitioners in the Nebraska farming community.

The conscious seven-year-old was moaning and agitated, so one of the doctors lifted him bodily by shoulders and knees to carry him to the X-ray room. Styner noted scant regard for his son's unsupported head or painful neck, either of which might be fractured. A few minutes later the medic emerged to declare cheerfully that the skull was intact. Was the spine OK? Blank look. It hadn't been looked at. Nor had anything else, so at this point the orthopaedic surgeon's relief at reaching the hospital disintegrated. In fact it turned to despair. Another motionless son was having his laceration sewn but there was no prioritising; no systematic physical examination and no airway protection despite unconsciousness. Nothing to keep them safe while their mother lay dead in a field.

By 4 a.m. Styner was in panic mode. Given the lack of informed help, he called his practice partner in Lincoln to explain the situation but in the meantime, a search aircraft from South Dakota had picked up the crashed aircraft's locator beacon. A helicopter piloted by one of Styner's old patients set off to find them and having done so, the Lincoln Air National Guard were asked to retrieve the injured family and bring them back to the city hospital 110 miles away.

The family arrived at the helipad in Lincoln at 8 am almost fourteen hours after the crash. The emergency room physician, Ron Craig, and Styner's own surgical colleagues were waiting for them with the operating theatres kept available in readiness. Fortunately everyone recovered, though the two unconscious children remained so for a week. It took many months for the emotional scars to heal. Styner was deeply troubled by the treatment they received that night. He commented 'When I can provide better care in a field with no resources than I received at the rural hospital, there is something wrong with the system. And the system has to be changed.' He didn't blame the staff as individuals; he simply lamented the fact that, as doctors who were expected to treat the injured, they had had no training. Their 'best efforts' were simply not good enough.

The established Advanced Cardiac Life Support course had been developed by the Lincoln Cardiologist Steve Carvith, together with their Mobile Heart Team who retrieved patients in shock after myocardial infarction. Logically, Styner and Craig liaised with one of the heart team nurses, Jodie Bechtel, to ascertain how a similar education process for trauma care could be rolled out in the region. Between them they came up with the Advanced Trauma Life Support course, widely abbreviated to ATLS. So successful was the concept that in 1982 another Lincoln heart team nurse, Irene Hughes, was taken on to manage a nationwide ATLS programme for the American College of Surgeons.

Perhaps the most valuable and uncontroversial contribution of ATLS was the ABC process of cardiopulmonary resuscitation adopted as the best method to prioritise interventions. What treatable problem was likely to kill the victim first? That was a

THE AMERICAN WAY

blocked airway (A), either from facial or neck injuries, swallowing the tongue or aspiration of vomit. Lack of oxygen rapidly damages the brain and head injuries in particular are beset by airway problems. Next, if the patient is physically unable to breathe (B), it's important to do that for them. Lastly, C stood for circulation. Should the patient lose a significant amount of blood or if their heart stops, that needs urgent help by transfusion or cardiac massage, or restoration of heart rhythm in order to distribute oxygen to the tissues.

This was protocol-driven medicine aimed at making the patient safe by fixing one problem at a time in sequence. This superseded looking at the patient as a whole, making a diagnosis, then going back to initiate treatment. At the time, it was the subject of much controversy but emerged as appropriate for life-threatening situations. I followed the guidelines on many occasions in my career both in the hospital and by the roadside.

The original ATLS course was field tested in Auburn, Nebraska, in 1978 and included a hands-on surgical skills room using live, anaesthetised dogs. I personally didn't like that. By the time I attended the course myself it had been rolled out throughout the United States but without using animals. What Styner and his co-workers conceived as an educational opportunity for rural Nebraska rapidly became a course for the world and a flagship for the military. Originally intended just for surgeons, the ATLS protocols were soon adapted for emergency room physicians, paramedics and nurses. But not everyone was happy with it, particularly the influence it had on clear fluid infusion in the pre-hospital setting. Least of all Howard Champion.

THE TRAUMA CHRONICLES

Howard eventually negotiated a shift in administrative control of pre-hospital care from the ATLS driven fire service to MedStar. As he told me on that first visit, 'if you give somebody a tool to play with,' referring to intravenous cannulas and bags of fluid, 'it's difficult to take it away. So I instituted the 'load and go' policy with no drips for journey times that were less than twenty minutes. We got the message across but it was a struggle.' The main area of conflict was with the emergency care physicians who found their trauma practice disappearing as the MedStar network spread throughout Maryland. In contrast, one senior police officer remarked 'Champion has single-handedly reduced the murder rate in the District of Columbia.'

My training in America had come to an end. The following morning I would board a jumbo jet and fly back to London. What I wished for most from the next couple of hours besides a last steak and bottle of Merlot, was to watch Champion's team take on a polytrauma case. I wasn't disappointed. Just as soon as he greeted me in the foyer of the Capital's largest teaching hospital, his pager went off. It was a code yellow alert warning of the arrival of a MedStar helicopter from the Washington DC beltway now closed by a high speed motor accident. When we reached the unit, the 'chopper' was descending onto the helipad just 20 yards from the emergency entrance. There were nine doctors and nurses waiting to receive the patient including a staff anaesthetist and the on call trauma surgeon. The others were residents in training from the Walter Reed Army Hospital and Bethesda Naval Hospital.

Receiving the injured woman on the helipad were the 'hot unload' team comprised of a trauma resuscitation

144

THE AMERICAN WAY

nurse and a respiratory therapist with the responsibility of securing the airway and breathing. Once in the department, her blood pressure was checked in both arms in case of an aortic injury, then wide bore intravenous lines were deftly inserted into neck and groin veins. As she was put to sleep, paralysed and intubated, an exploratory catheter was inserted through the wall of her swollen belly which immediately drained blood. Rapid confirmation of serious abdominal injuries.

That whole process took less than ten minutes, after which the victim was wheeled through into an operating theatre no more than 20 feet from the reception bay. After moving her from trolley to the operating table, an overhead X-ray machine took a chest X-ray to rule out unsuspected injuries. And as a routine precaution, the whole of the torso was prepped with antiseptic solution and draped in such a way that the abdominal incision could be extended into the chest should that prove necessary. For me the efficiency of the rescue process was mind boggling. Poetry in motion compared to the nursery rhymes we endured in Britain. Yet the process was initiated from Birmingham, England. From an innovative centre destined for closure.

Within thirty minutes of the helicopter landing the abdomen was opened down the midline. As is often the case, blood slopped out over the drapes with the source of bleeding not readily apparent. So several large linen packs were pushed into the left upper quadrant around the spleen, then the right upper quadrant around the liver and lastly down into the pelvis. The objective was to put pressure on the bleeding sites, soak up free blood, and encourage clotting within the damaged organs. Meanwhile, the anaesthetist transfused uncross-matched

145

blood to nudge up the pressure to tolerable levels. Clearly there is little point pouring in the precious resource while it continues to leak from a damaged blood vessel. That is equivalent to pouring water into a bucket when there is a gaping hole at the bottom. The higher the blood pressure the faster the leak. In patients you need a surgeon to close holes, not well-meaning others to piss into a leaky pot.

As the linen coverings soaked up the blood and damped down the bleeding, scrutiny of the chest X-ray showed the diaphragm to be pushed upwards on the right side, reinforcing the suspicion of a ruptured liver. So the packs were gently removed from the pelvis and spleen first. By exclusion, the liver had to be the problem as was expected from the blood loss. When the sloppy packs were gradually peeled away a huge and potentially lethal laceration was exposed. This was closed carefully with a large curved needle and catgut stitches passed deep into the fragile tissue. More packs were then used to cover the repair exerting more pressure to damp down the oozing. As those of you who eat liver will appreciate, to sew the offal and tighten the stitches is not easy. They can easily tear through making matters worse. Of course, there was nothing special about shoving in packs and sewing up tears in the liver. I had done that on numerous occasions as a registrar in Cambridge. It was the ruthless regimentation of the whole rescue that impressed me and made me sad for what patients had to endure in the NHS.

That case of liver trauma embodied the whole rationale for preserving the body's own blood clotting mechanisms and not destroying that vital process with litres of

THE AMERICAN WAY

cold, clear fluid. The message is simple. Surgeons need nature on our side, otherwise the chances of success are diminished.

After thirty minutes of restrained waiting, all bleeding had stopped. With that, the abdominal cavity was carefully washed out with salt solution and closed up. The twenty-five year old was admitted to intensive care for twenty-four hours and as I learned back in England she had gone home after five days in hospital having arrived moribund with haemorrhagic shock. Lucky lady. No one had asked her permission to operate or whether she could pay or not. MedStar was a massively impressive system that saved lives through awesome efficiency. But now, my time in the US was over and I had to return to Britain. I needed to fit in again with 'socialised medicine'. More and more that was becoming a euphemism for what I termed 'second hand shop' healthcare.

Needless Deaths

If you want happiness for an hour, take a nap. If
you want happiness for a day, go fishing. If you
want yearlong happiness, inherit a fortune. It you
want happiness for lifetime, help someone else.

Ancient Chinese proverb

The transition to working in London was predictably difficult and frustrating. In Alabama, then at MedStar in Washington, I learned to push the envelope to benefit the sick. Yet while we had great doctors and nurses back home, the organisation of the NHS revolved around cost containment. Saving money trumped saving lives, and I was perpetually disturbed by that. My personal objectives remained focused on finding a teaching hospital post in cardiac surgery, but in comparison with the United States, even my time at Great Ormond Street and the Hammersmith Hospitals was a disappointment. But saying so was never going to boost my career prospects.

I'd been back just a few weeks when I received a desperately miserable call from the mother of an old school friend. She was an intelligent woman, a lawyer, who was beside herself with grief. Earlier that evening her son's motorcycle had been nudged off the road by a lorry and smashed into a lamppost at high speed. He was now in the casualty department of a general hospital in the north of England and his parents were informed that he was unlikely to survive. That was the only information that they were given. In despair, she wondered whether I would call to enquire what injuries he had sustained and what was it that heralded the dismal prognosis. The caller hadn't responded to questions and she was troubled by his defensive tone.

What else could I do. Obviously I felt obliged to probe, but from experience I knew the call to be unwelcome. Unnecessary interference at a difficult time. The dialogue went as follows:

'Hello, could I have a word with Sister in Charge please?' Then came the curt response which I fully anticipated

'I'm sorry she's busy with a patient. I'm the receptionist, can I help you?'

I said 'I'm a surgeon in London and gather that a personal friend is with you after a traffic accident. Would someone be prepared to have a word with me about it?' The line went quiet for a few seconds, then came 'Sister's with him now, but I'll see if someone else will talk to you.' Then I waited. And waited. And waited for a very long time.

Eventually, a male voice said 'Hello, I'm the senior house officer. Can I help you?'

'Hopefully you can, I'm enquiring about the motorcyclist whom I believe is in the Emergency room.' Again a pause.

'Yes, I've been looking after him and I should be there now.' I felt told off. 'He's not doing well I'm afraid. His abdomen is distended and the chest X-ray doesn't look good. A widened mediastinum.' That's the middle bit between the lungs on each side. 'He may have ruptured his aorta.'

So I politely asked who was going to sort it all out and in what order? A torn aorta and intra-abdominal bleeding is a worrying combination. I was not reassured by the reply.

'We've asked the general surgeons to come and look at him but they're still busy in theatre.'

'So how is he now?' I asked with an air of irritation.

'To be honest I think we're going to lose him. We've asked the regional cardiothoracic unit if they'll take him but they won't let us transfer him until the belly is sorted out.' I tried to press him further but could tell that he wanted an end to the conversation.

'What is his blood pressure, if you don't mind me asking?'

'About 60 systolic,' he grumbled in resignation, so I asked whether he was receiving blood to help with that. Apparently he'd been given more than six litres of clear fluid. The blood was being cross matched.

'Look, has a consultant seen him?' I pressed. 'His mother's a solicitor.' That comment really didn't help either but sometimes it focuses minds. The house officer's glib response – 'there's an anaesthetic consultant who's been asked to come but he's still in theatre too!'

An 'oh shit' moment crashed over me like a wave. My school friend was clearly about to die with no realistic efforts mounted to save him. It's rather obvious, as we have said. If there is a hole near the bottom of a bucket water will pour out of it and the greater the head of pressure above, the faster it will leak. You can keep pouring more water into the top but it will still piss out of the bottom. The human circulation is no different. Damage to a major blood vessel or organ will bleed but as the blood pressure falls the bleeding slows, offering

THE TRAUMA CHRONICLES

the body's natural clotting mechanisms a chance to plug the defect. To pour in fluid at room temperature that does not carry oxygen simply perpetuates the blood loss and dilutes the clotting factors. What's more, the lowering of temperature and oxygen carrying capacity simply exacerbate the metabolic derangement of shock—a risk in itself. So if you have a leak in your bucket close the bloody hole. That's what surgeons do. That's not what was happening in that distant casualty department. Nothing was being done to help. On the contrary. Inexperienced staff were presiding over the natural history of untreated injuries.

What would I say to that poor mother? Should I be kind and say 'everything possible is being done to save your son, but despite their best efforts...' Or did I owe her the truth? That he might as well have been left to die by the roadside. This wasn't rural Nebraska but the industrial heartlands of northern England in 1982. Regrettably, it was the same in most hospitals in the UK. Even my great training hospital, Addenbrooke's in Cambridge, had its weaknesses. It had great general, brain and orthopaedic surgeons but the chest surgeons were many miles away in the countryside. So who would repair a torn aorta? I remembered that futile attempt in the accident department one winter's afternoon when Sister McDougall was in charge. The poor student was bleeding profusely and I failed miserably.

So why wouldn't our NHS, the 'envy of the world' get its act together? Each year there were 20,000 or more fatalities from injury in Britain and trauma was the most common cause of death in young people. Moreover, for every mortality two survivors were left with permanent disabilities providing huge financial implications for society in general. But the NHS was blatantly a political organisation with its own agenda. Consider the frustrating attempts by numerous medical organisations to introduce seat belt legislation. This was collectively opposed by both the Conservative Government and the Labour opposition on thirteen separate attempts before a watered down proposal was eventually accepted in July 1981. Even then, the law only came into practice in 1983. Given the compliance of 90% of drivers the result was a 29% reduction in fatalities and a 30% decrease overall in life-threatening injuries. Perhaps the US should accept appropriate fire arms legislation to do the same!

Soon after I had returned the mother's call she heard that they had lost him. After that debacle I decided to make an effort to do something about it. Perhaps it would have been wiser to wait until I had my precious consultancy post but I had no idea how long that might take. To begin with, the safest route was to write articles about my experiences for medical journals. One of the first was in the Lancet describing a technique that I had devised for rapid blood transfusion in exsanguinating patients. Then I described a couple of surgical reconstructive techniques in the chest where I used grafts of diaphragm muscle. Both papers were published in prestigious American journals. One thing led to another, resulting in my first modest textbook entitled 'Wound Care' published in 1985. That was followed a couple of years later by 'Trauma, Pathogenesis and Treatment' lavishly illustrated with gore from an ever increasing portfolio of my own trauma cases.

I wasn't the only surgeon in the UK to complain bitterly about the NHS's management of life-threatening

THE TRAUMA CHRONICLES

injuries. During my medical school days, a Government Accident Services Review had suggested wide ranging improvements including a three tier treatment system according to injury severity. Tier one was intended to be a general practitioner-led service for minor injuries in the community. More serious tier two cases would be taken to district general hospital casualty department for assessment and triage. These were renamed Accident and Emergency Departments and given that broken bones featured more frequently than internal organ damage, the orthopaedic surgeons were placed in the driving seat. In tier three, those who needed specialist expertise and resources including brain and chest operations would be secondarily referred to the major teaching hospitals. Inevitably, this system proved seriously wanting if for no other reason than inter-hospital transfer of the critically injured took hours and often proved fatal.

A subsequent study showed that senior medical cover at the front door was practically non-existent, with desperately poor standards of care. Sadly that was already readily apparent to me from my own misadventures as a young man. But in those days, the NHS remained an unquestionable religion. People didn't have to pay at the door so what happened on the other side of the portal was rarely scrutinised. And death was cheap.

NHS planners made the critical miscalculation that only the seriously sick or injured would find their way to the fancy tier two Accident and Emergency centres once the term 'casualty department' was abandoned. On the contrary, they were inundated with minor injuries, general medical cases and many problems of a social or psychiatric nature. Orthopaedic surgeons were the last group interested in handling this workload and stayed in their operating theatres. Nursing sisters, like my own dear Sarah, were left in charge and frankly did a much better job in organising the junior doctors.

It was in the late 1970s, as I trained in surgery, that the government announced that thirty-two large city based Accident Departments should be home to a new medical specialty designated as 'Accident and Emergency Medicine,' a role which persists today. This concept did make a substantial difference by placing senior medical staff in the reception area of those nominated hospitals and improving departmental organisation overall. Yet major obstacles remained in the readiness to treat serious internal injuries that could only be saved by surgery. The United States were gradually getting to grips with the situation, we weren't, hence my adventures from the base at Harefield.

Champion was collaborating on the research side with the trauma surgery pioneer, Donald Trunkey of San Francisco. Trunkey collected a huge bank of data on deaths from injury and recognised a distinct trimodal pattern. The major peak occurred within minutes of the accident or assault frequently before hospital admission. Those victims, accounting for half of the total, died through catastrophic injuries to the brain, heart or major blood vessels which proved rapidly fatal. At the other end of the spectrum, in a third peak, were hospital deaths from complications of surgery or sepsis in the lungs or blood stream. Again, little could be done to prevent these poor outcomes.

The realm where a substantial improvement could be made was in the middle peak, where effective early management proved vital for survival. Many second peak patients had head injuries and, having been rendered unconscious, they died from remediable obstruction to their airways and breathing. Others had internal bleeding from damaged organs but with the potential to be rescued by rapid transit to a skilled surgical team. Their deaths were coined 'failure to rescue,' an important descriptive term that I subsequently applied in cardiac surgery. Trunkey's claim was that many who died should have been saved by better pre-hospital and Emergency room care.

To illustrate the benefits of a well organised system, he made a direct comparison of outcomes following motor vehicle accidents when the patients were taken to either the San Francisco County major trauma centre or to the multiple general hospitals in neighbouring Orange County. The results were quite staggering. In Orange County, one third of head injury patients and two thirds of those with chest or abdominal injuries were deemed to have died unnecessarily. Contrast that with one single potentially avoidable death in San Francisco County. Indeed, the US military had already shown the value of early aggressive intervention in the Vietnam War where the helicopters carried army medics tasked with clearing a blocked airway or giving uncross-matched blood transfusion to those exsanguinating from penetrating wounds.

It was then that a number of major disasters heightened public awareness in Britain. Certainly the bombing of the Grand Hotel in Brighton during the Conservative Party Conference served to focus the minds of the politicians. How could multiple injuries of the head, torso and limbs be treated adequately by junior doctors or physicians? Could bog standard district general hospitals ever reduce mortality rates in the multiply

156

NEEDLESS DEATHS

injured? After all, polytrauma accounted for only 2% of the Emergency Department's workload and specialised surgeons don't grow on trees. When needed urgently they would usually be committed to their routine work.

For me, trauma was a side-line that I enjoyed through its unpredictability and rich rewards. But for most cardiothoracic surgeons it was an irritating and sometimes intimidating diversion from what they were trained for. So as my books and papers became visible on the subject, I was pleased to be asked to participate in a Royal College of Surgeons Working Party on trauma. At last the surgeons themselves wanted to improve things and I was excited to be a part of it as a mere trainee. Albeit a very experienced trainee.

The prestigious committee was chaired by Miles Irving, the dynamic Professor of Surgery from Manchester who had previously worked with the victims from a number of major incidents in London. One of his many anecdotes typified the view of that bygone era. As a young consultant at St Bartholomew's Hospital in the city of London, he was in the casualty department triaging the many bleeding and choking victims of a bombing at the Old Bailey. The matron of the hospital walked through the department, stopping briefly to say 'I see you're very busy Mr Irving. I'd love to stop and help you but I have a committee meeting in a few minutes.' I thought that summed things up rather well. Important people in the NHS discuss, not act. Bugger the suffering hordes when there are dignitaries waiting to talk, and decisions about budgets to be made.

Peter London, Howard's old boss and the doyen of the Birmingham Accident Hospital, was another trauma committee member, so I was honoured to be

157

amongst them. Against the depressing background of complacency, our remit was to establish the facts surrounding deaths from injury in Britain then propose solutions for the deficiencies. Since we all had busy day jobs, the college employed a full time research fellow for two years to gather the information.

First, we made a detailed assessment of the circumstances of one thousand trauma deaths from eleven coroners districts covering a range of major cities, towns and rural areas. Of those patients, almost half perished before they reached hospital, the remainder died subsequently following initial assessment and treatment. Notably, the majority were young people between the ages of 20 to 29 years. Full details of their management and autopsy findings were considered by the committee members and the question posed: had this patient been admitted to a fully-staffed and equipped US-style trauma centre might their death have been prevented? The simple answer, yes or no, was required, after which the death was recorded as preventable if at least three of four assessors deemed it to be so.

The data showed that, at minimum, one third of the hospital deaths should never have occurred. At a conservative estimate, more than 300 of the patients should have survived. Sad, particularly if it happened to be your son or daughter. One third of these were head injuries with intracranial bleeding amenable to surgery. The remainder followed bleeding into the chest or abdomen which would not have caused death with a timely operation. 'Failure to rescue' is the appropriate term. Indeed, 79% of those who could definitely have been saved by surgery simply didn't get it. They received the ABC of drips, fluids and breathing tubes but that doesn't stop bleeding. Think hole in the bucket. Without surgery, fluid infusion makes things worse. No red blood cells, no oxygen.

One of the main issues we highlighted was the sheer lack of experience in those on the front line. This, together with absence of executive decision making or failure to recognise a life-threatening diagnosis. Twenty-two shattered livers were missed, twelve ruptured spleens and eighteen torn and bleeding lungs. Of those with head injuries, the type of brain haemorrhage that even I had operated upon successfully as a trainee remained unrecognised. And precious few of the dead patients had been seen by a consultant. In other words, the care received by many was a shameful shambles, yet accepted without challenge by our NHS. Until our investigation that is.

The final report indicated that, by conservative estimates, there were at least 2,500 wholly preventable deaths from injury in England each year, most occurring through poor treatment overall and failure to operate on bleeding. Consequently, we made strong recommendation that the NHS should study and follow the example of North America by establishing a network of dedicated trauma centres to treat major injuries. In contrast, the existing general Accident and Emergency Departments should continue to manage cuts, bruises and straightforward limb fractures together with their medical and psychiatric workload. It was pretty obvious really. After all, that whole US initiative had arisen from the Birmingham Accident Hospital model which was dispensed with less than ten years after Peter London retired.

As an official Royal College of Surgeon's report highlighting needless deaths in young people, we

THE TRAUMA CHRONICLES

triggered widespread debate in the media. And the usual crap ensued. Naysayers deemed the concept too expensive for a state funded health system. Death is cheap. As I've said already, cost containment was repeatedly prioritised over saving lives. Miles Irving's retort was that, given a debacle that accounts for one percent of our gross national product, the expense of creating regional trauma centres would undoubtedly be small in comparison. Obvious again but not persuasive enough in the Department of Health.

The next excuse was that the US model was untried in the UK. It seemed that the Birmingham Accident Hospital was sufficiently far from the metropolis not to have been noticed, but surely a pilot scheme was indicated at the very least! The next absurd suggestion was to simply double the number of Accident and Emergency consultants. That completely missed the point. They are trained as physicians not surgeons. They can resuscitate but don't operate. What we desperately lacked was trained trauma surgeons on the front line. Surgeons that operate within the chest, abdomen and skull, not just on broken bones. Close the hole in the bucket, don't keep pouring fluid into the top of it.

Other sceptics voiced the possibility of a negative effect on morale in existing Accident and Emergency Departments should their handful of major trauma cases be diverted elsewhere. As Miles annotated in one of his lectures, 'I find this an amazing suggestion. Do patients really have to be treated in less than ideal circumstances just to maintain the morale of a hospital department?' What's more, I was fully aware from Sister Sarah that nothing destroyed morale faster at the front door than a total cock up precipitating the death of a young patient.

The question then arose as to the maintenance of competence in our district general hospitals should major disaster happen in proximity. Would a downgraded Accident and Emergency Department be able to cope? Were they coping now, was the obvious question. Could things get any worse? But actually the real answer was that, by and large, major incidents are usually dealt with admirably by general hospitals. Why? Because everything else stops. The whole hospital responds to an influx of multiple casualties by turning themselves into a temporary trauma centre. All consultant surgeons and anaesthetists are alerted rapidly and commit to the rescue efforts with their teams. It is the involvement of an experienced surgical team that makes the difference, not the buildings or equipment that conventionally comprise a trauma centre.

It wasn't just a lacklustre performance on hospital admission that warranted improvement. The incidence of pre-hospital trauma deaths varied widely from 20% to 80% in different coroners' districts. Much of this variation reflected the time it was taking to bring the patient in, particularly over long distances. In that context, we knew that rapid transit by helicopter was making a difference in Germany and the United States. Yet in Britain it was premature to introduce that degree of sophistication until the services at the receiving end were able to cope.

By the time the report was released I was awarded a prestigious consultant post in Oxford, with the remit to build a new cardiothoracic centre to fill the gap between London and Birmingham, Bristol to Cambridge. I had no doubt that I was given the job thanks to testimonials from London cardiologists who confirmed that I could operate. As one of the world's premier academic centres, Oxford wanted the usual adult heart and lung surgery practice but had ambitions for a congenital heart unit too. That meant operating on all comers from premature babies with deformed hearts to adults with inherited cardiac problems. Thanks to Dr Kirklin and colleagues, I could do all that and was fortunately the only applicant, including scores of existing consultants, who had sufficient experience to take it on. An intimidating task bearing in mind that there were no senior colleagues to call upon. But at least I had Sarah to talk to. We married before I took up the post and, impoverished as we were, we lived on site in dismal hospital accommodation. For a prolonged period, I would be the only cardiothoracic surgeon for a huge region, yet I thrived on the autonomy and, inevitably, every major chest trauma case came my way. So I gave more lectures, collected more photographs of the cases, and wrote more papers on the subject. There was no downtime and for the first three years I was constantly on call, day and night.

As it happened, a somewhat dramatic case presented itself during my first week at the John Radcliffe Hospital. My brand new pager alerted me at 08.00 and requested my immediate presence in the accident department. I guess most hospitals would have put out a call for the cardiothoracic registrar or senior house officer, but there were none. I stood alone as the whole department at that stage.

The emergency room was otherwise quiet but with frenetic activity around one cubicle where the curtains were drawn. There was Sister in Charge, rushing in with bags of dextrose solution from the fridge, which

NEEDLESS DEATHS

suggested a degree of blood loss in the case, but when I pulled open the drapes the problem was readily apparent. Supine on the trolley was an agitated young man already stripped to the waist. He was pale as a sheet, staring intently at the overhead strip lights to divert his gaze from a large oriental dagger protruding from the centre of his chest. The ominous instrument was in perpetual motion like a metronome. While sister suspended the bag of fluid from the drip stand, a young casualty officer with a distinct air of panic was vainly attempting to insert an intravenous cannula into a vein in the lad's forearm. Difficult because the patient was convulsing with fear and the doctor's hands were trembling with anxiety. Not a scene that inspired me with confidence.

The executive functioning department of my own frontal lobes took over. First question, 'have you measured the blood pressure yet?'

'Yes it's 100/70 but his pulse rate is up to 118.' Sister said.

'Just relax then,' I said calmly. 'Do nothing for now. Perhaps you would call theatre 5 for me. I'm meant to have a case in there.' Then after a pregnant pause, I said 'please.' After all it was Oxford.

I turned to the patient and sternly told him to keep still, close his eyes and think of something pleasant while I put the drip in myself. He was of slim build and, from the prominent distended veins in his neck, I could tell that the sac around his heart was filled with blood. This was the standard cardiac stab wound presentation for those fortunate enough to reach hospital. Had the knife been withdrawn he would have died swiftly. That blade was plugging the hole.

THE TRAUMA CHRONICLES

Sister returned to say she had theatre 5 on the line. I asked them to put the day's first customer on hold as I would be pushing round a young man with a knife in his heart. But not to send the poor valve replacement patient back to the ward. The stab wound wouldn't take long. They clearly thought the new surgeon was bonkers, but actually it didn't take long. I ran the saw up the breast bone with the knife in place. Then gently distracted the two halves to visualise the blue distended sac around his heart. Zipping that open with dissecting scissors, I sucked out the liquid blood then withdraw the blade under direct vision. I could then place a finger over the defect and stitch it carefully. He really didn't need any fluid or blood transfusion. Remember, close the hole in the bucket first. Then decide whether to fill it up again. He didn't need to go to intensive care afterwards. He woke up immediately and had supper on the ward.

This was a good case to kick off my consultant career and I soon heard what was said about me. 'Shit, he's a cool customer.' Cool perhaps, but for me it was easy to close a wound in the right ventricle. Three carefully placed nylon stitched did the job. Anyway, why should I be anxious about it? It wasn't me on the operating table. Psychopath.

The disturbed young man was a student of African and Oriental Studies at Brasenose College, which kindly offered me dining rights. Anxiety was his problem, particularly at exam time, and on this occasion the strain had been too much for him. So, after a sleepless night, he took the knife—bought on a trip to Zanzibar—and aimed it carefully at his own heart. He succeeded in penetrating the chest wall but, apart from the searing pain, he felt no difference. So, leaning against the wall

NEEDLESS DEATHS

of his college room he thrust again. That hurt more and he felt faint—perhaps through bleeding, possibly from the shock of it all. When he still didn't die in desperation he had another go. The knife went deeper still but he remained in control of his faculties.

Having failed in his determined quest he left his room and walked to the porters lodge with the protruding implement visible to all. Fortunately, most of the students were still in bed or having breakfast in the hall. As he staggered into the lodge the doorman, who had yet to have his bacon sandwich, fainted and banged his head on the desk. For expediency, the ambulance brought them both into hospital together. And I'm pleased to report that they both recovered uneventfully. The student was really grateful to have survived, as abortive suicides usually are. So much so that, for many years, he sent me a regular update on his happy life. And I still have that knife. I thought it best to keep it away from him.

How was it possible to quantify the risks of a patient dying from their injuries so that we could justify a realistic comparison between Britain and the US? Howard and I were still in contact and I knew he was working on a system of Injury Severity Scores. These were based on a points system which reflected the magnitude of injury to the internal organs and skeleton but factored in the patient's age, degree of frailty through comorbid medical problems, and even the degree of metabolic derangement at the time of hospital admission. This scoring system provided a statistically based approach to predicting mortality that was eventually adopted by our own Department of Health for further studies on preventable deaths. Then, under Miles Irving's influence, a consortium of hospitals in the North West of England received a government grant to prospectively collect and analyse information on deaths from injury beginning in 1989. This became the first UK Major Trauma Outcome Study. Hopefully we were finally getting somewhere.

Using information equivalent to that collected by our American colleagues, Irving and the Hope Hospital group in Salford became the only British contributors to Champion's US Trauma Outcome Study in Washington. At least we had an unbiased objective method to compare our NHS hospital performance with the well-resourced equivalent in what we used to call 'the colonies.' When the study reported its findings, the news was not good.

The information was derived from thirty-three front line NHS hospitals reporting on 15,000 seriously injured patients. It took one fifth of them more than an hour to reach an accident department. Then, more than half were met and resuscitated by a very junior doctor. Fewer than half with injuries requiring urgent surgery reached an operating theatre within two hours. Once there, the vast majority were operated upon by a trainee surgeon, not a consultant. As a result, the death rates for the sickest were markedly greater than in an American centre.

One glaringly obvious cause for excessive mortality was that the various surgical specialties needed to collaborate in polytrauma were rarely located in the same hospital. It was the same in Oxford. The brain surgeons were in the grand old Radcliffe Infirmary in the city centre. The general and cardiothoracic surgeons worked at the John Radcliffe Hospital, the new acute health campus by the ring road. And, needless to say, the specialist orthopaedic and plastic surgeons were in separate buildings in a different part of town. Great hospitals and splendid surgeons but they were dispersed throughout the city by poor organisation. A seriously injured patient might need all of those specialists so what were the chances of them coming together in a reasonable time frame? Zero.

The study findings again confirmed that critically injured patients received very poor care in the NHS and many died unnecessarily. Under mounting pressure and at the instigation of our College of Surgeons committee members, the Department of Health finally agreed to fund a pilot US-style trauma centre in Stoke-on-Trent in the Midlands. This served a population of half a million covered by a single coroner's office at a time when there was fierce debate as to whether more help should be offered in the pre-hospital setting. So the first thing Stoke did was to look into that area.

Once again their findings were interesting but disappointing. Amongst 409 trauma deaths, 152 occurred before reaching hospital in patients averaging forty-two years of age. Using similar criteria to our College of Surgeons' preventable death studies, at least 60 of the 152 patients could have been saved, fifty-one by basic attention to an obstructed airway. The simple conclusion was that first aid at the accident site could save many young lives. But how far should those efforts be taken?

The findings applied principally to the unconscious patient with head injuries who swallowed their tongue or were unable to cough and clear their own breathing tubes. Aside from A and B, was it justified to waste time at the site for other interventions particularly when the patient was bleeding? That debate was reverberating around the US who were ten years or more ahead of us.

And despite the Stoke-on-Trent pilot, the news had not improved for Britain.

In 1992, a National Audit Office report again highlighted many serious deficiencies in NHS Accident and Emergency Departments stating that widespread improvements were necessary. That same year, the British Orthopaedic Association presented a detailed review of trauma services in 263 NHS hospitals which documented the lack of both staffing and equipment. They concluded that our efforts on behalf of the injured had not kept pace with advances in technology or strategy. They urged, as we did, the need for regional trauma centres where senior medical staff would involve themselves with those who faced imminent death. Not a difficult concept to understand. Five years later, the same group published a comparative study that highlighted inferior NHS outcomes in comparison with the Swiss, German and US systems. And so it went on. When would anyone take notice?

Perhaps the most devastating of published investigations was by the UK National Confidential Enquiry into Post-operative Deaths which found that 60% of trauma patients who perished after surgery had not received adequate care. What an indictment of any health care system. A medico-legal minefield with potentially ruinous compensation costs. The recommendations were clear. The dismal treatment of the injured by NHS hospitals needed radical reform. This should occur through the roll out of regional trauma centres with a consultant and back up team present day and night to triage and expedite care.

It had been fifteen years since our Royal College of Surgeons report had recommended the same. So many

NEEDLESS DEATHS

patients died needlessly in the interim. Worse still it wasn't just the injured that we were losing needlessly. I was well familiar with circulatory support devices used to save dying heart attack patients in the US and Europe. The NHS wouldn't fund them even in cardiac surgery centres.

'Scoop and run' or 'Stay and play'

> Everybody is a genius. But if you judge a fish by
> its ability to climb a tree it will live its whole life
> believing that it is stupid.
>
> Albert Einstein

You may assume from my comments that I have reservations about pre-hospital care. It should go without saying that I have the highest regard for ambulance staff and paramedics who do a difficult job on a daily basis. In fact, I would regularly invite them into the operating theatre to watch their case if they had the time. I gave talks for them and recommended the job to many people including my own son. But before the NHS even moved from pre-hospital 'first aid' measures to so called 'advanced life support,' evidence emerged from the US that invasive care was often unnecessary and, in some patients, caused worse outcomes.

As we have said, bleeding from internal organs is a time-sensitive, life-threatening issue that can only be remedied by surgery. Therefore, rapid transport to a hospital capable of delivering that option is imperative if unnecessary deaths are to be avoided. 'Scoop and run' is the relevant term. It's what the ambulance service did in the old days as matter of course. Sure, the airways would be cleared first and the neck stabilised. Assisted breathing was by a valved air bag and face mask, not through a tube in the windpipe. More time dependent procedures like putting up drips and passing endotracheal tubes were not considered—this is 'stay and play.' Of course there is no definitive answer between 'scoop and run' versus 'stay and play.' Every injured patient has individual needs so generalised protocols will always let down a proportion of them. That's why some affluent systems send doctors to an accident scene, but when that is the case they invariably find a reason to intervene.

What particularly troubled me as a surgeon was the ATLS guideline of administering two litres of clear fluid to injured patients whose blood pressure had fallen. Firstly, it was impossible to know what internal injuries they had and second, vasovagal shock will drop pressure in the absence of blood loss. Estimating blood pressure in the pre-hospital setting is open to misinterpretation. It was generally taught that if a pulse cannot be felt at the wrist the pressure must have fallen below 80 mm Hg. And should only the carotid artery pulse be palpable in the neck it must be down to 60 mm Hg. But all my patients on the heart-lung machine have an average pressure between 60-70 mm Hg. It's flow that is important, not pressure. There are better ways to monitor shock from bleeding.

One way is to think about scores in a game of tennis. Love – 15 – 30 – 40 – game over. When 15% of the blood volume is lost, around 750 mls, that is the same as a blood donor session and doesn't change the pressure. Yet it will increase the heart rate to around 100 beats per minute and the patient is likely to be anxious. If 30% or 1.5 litres of the circulating blood is lost, the pressure falls to around 100 mm Hg with a heart rate climbing above 100 bpm and the patient starts to breathe faster.

'SCOOP AND RUN' OR 'STAY AND PLAY'

But there is still no reason to panic or transfuse. Not until the patient reaches 40 to love having bled more than 2 litres and with absent pulses at the wrist and groin, is he in trouble. The respiratory rate then exceeds 30 breaths per minute and the kidneys stop producing urine. He becomes confused and lethargic which is not helped by using fluids that cannot carry oxygen. Trauma patients with altered mental state and circulatory collapse are at exceedingly high risk for death. Without blood transfusion and an operation to stop the bleeding quickly, it is game over.

So what are the consequences of pouring in salt or sugar solution in an attempt to raise blood pressure? In the US they referred to it as the lethal triad. First, the blood's ability to clot and plug holes is destroyed. Next, fluid at ambient temperature automatically lowers body temperature with the adverse effects of hypothermia. Lastly, elevation of blood pressure before the injuries are repaired causes clot dislodgement and further bleeding. None of that made my job any easier.

Let's reconsider the merits of scoop and run versus stay and play on the basis of actual clinical experience, rather than my own gut feelings. We know that half of trauma deaths occur rapidly at the scene from unsurvivable injuries that are not influenced by pre-hospital care. It is those patients who die in hospital within twenty-four hours of their injuries that conceivably could benefit, but do they and to what extent?

The ATLS trained responders, whether doctors or paramedics, have a range of procedures available to them. If we follow the ABC resuscitation algorithm they can provide definitive airway control with tracheal intubation, ventilate the patient with oxygen, insert a cannula into a vein to give fluids, and perform external cardiac massage for cardiac arrest. That initial portfolio was extended to inserting needles or drains through the chest wall or even opening the chest surgically in some circumstances. All this is done on the basis of cursory clinical examination, not as a result of the investigations available at short notice in hospitals.

While these pre-hospital interventions have theoretical advantages, the evidence supporting their effectiveness is limited and—on the contrary—may point to harm by prolonging the time to diagnosis and treatment. For those with a major but potentially survivable injury we do know that their odds of death increase by two to four per cent every minute before they reach an operating theatre or receive damage control resuscitation with blood transfusion.

In countries like France, where experienced doctors routinely attend accidents, some studies have shown on site rapid intubation of the windpipe—employing sedation and a muscle-paralysing agent—to improve survival for unconscious head injury patients and some with catastrophic chest injuries. But the same does not apply to the infusion of clear fluids in this setting. On the contrary, numerous published studies which compare basic life support measures with advanced life support techniques using fluid infusion have demonstrated an absence of benefit or even actual harm from the invasive approach. For instance, it has been shown repeatedly that patients with stab or gunshot wounds who receive advanced life support have worse survival rates.

A key head injury study comparing advanced life support provided by doctors using helicopter transport, versus basic life support given by paramedics in

'SCOOP AND RUN' OR 'STAY AND PLAY'

ambulances, showed no reduction in mortality by the former. Worryingly, another study from Pennsylvania that factored in the severity of injury demonstrated a fourfold greater risk of death for patients who underwent intubation of the windpipe at the accident site. There were reasons for that, one being that sedation and paralysis can induce cardiac arrest in trauma patients. It blunts the body's response to its own adrenaline release, drops the blood pressure and impairs the heart's contractility.

While efforts to intubate take time and are not always successful it is the physiological effects that are known to be damaging. There is a tendency to over ventilate which reduces the amount of carbon dioxide in the blood and reflexly reduces blood flow to an injured brain. In turn, positive pressure ventilation increases the pressure within the chest cavity which impedes the return of blood to the heart, and increases tension within the skull. While pre-hospital intubation itself may not be harmful the damaging effects of hyperventilation certainly are.

But back to fluids. With the advent of ATLS pre-hospital protocols, both doctors and paramedics believed it to be obligatory to insert an intravenous line on scene before setting off for the hospital. However this may prove difficult with average times taken between eight and twelve minutes. Time is one of the most critical aspects of trauma care so the performance of intravenous access or tracheal intubation must be weighed against the hazards of delay. In urban areas these interventions often take longer than the actual transport time.

Again we should resort to facts. In 2009 the US Eastern Association for the Surgery of Trauma scrutinised all available literature written in English since 1982 regarding pre-hospital fluid resuscitation for the injured patient. That amounted to 3,392 published research articles which included many thousands of patients. They concluded with two important findings. First there was no evidence that patients benefitted from clear fluid infusion in the pre-hospital setting. Then second, and critically, cannulation of a vein should never be attempted at the cost of delaying rapid transit to hospital.

There were just two situations when it was useful to have a cannula in place. The first was when drugs were needed to ensure safe insertion of a tracheal tube when airway problems were immediately life-threatening. The second was when blood was available for immediate transfusion on site in shocked patients. From a selfish standpoint I was repeatedly frustrated by having to perform major chest and blood vessel surgery on patients awash with fluid. They would always bleed more because their blood clotting factors were diluted and they were usually hypothermic and a metabolic mess, because the fluid used was well below body temperature.

By the mid-1990s, I was ensconced in Oxford which we had taken from the smallest to the second most productive cardiothoracic centre in the UK (after Cambridge). Just three surgeons were performing 1400 cardiac operations and I had launched the children's heart surgery programme. But now there was a new challenge. In tandem with surgeons in Houston, I was working on a new type of miniature artificial heart. This, I hoped, would evolve into a realistic alternative to heart transplants given that seat belt legislation

'SCOOP AND RUN' OR 'STAY AND PLAY'

had succeeded in driving down the numbers of fatally injured head injury patients from whom the organs were obtained.

In rare moments of downtime, I was collecting material for a lavishly illustrated textbook describing the compelling origins of my specialty. The motivation to write 'Landmarks in Cardiac Surgery' was derived from my career experiences in London and the US where I worked with or encountered many of the pioneers in their twilight years. Invariably I found their reckless ingenuity when operating on the beating heart both romantic and heroic. It just couldn't happen in the current era of risk management and accountability. Though few are aware of the fact, some of the earliest successes were in operations to remove bullets or shrapnel from the cardiac chambers during World War II. The remnants of the US military field hospital can still be found in the countryside near Oxford, where one dilapidated Nissen hut turned operating theatre remains.

During my impressionable school years, the legendary Christiaan Barnard performed the first human heart transplant in Cape Town. The donor was an unfortunate young woman, Denise Darvall who sustained a serious head injury when hit by a car driven by a drunken policeman. There was no definition of brain death and Barnard's assistants would only countenance removal of the heart when it had stopped beating. Tricky. The recipient, who would have never been regarded as suitable these days died a week later but news of the operation shocked the world to the same extent as the first moon landing. Barnard became a household name overnight. A rock star whose conjugal escapades led to divorce and eventually destroyed his professional reputation.

177

I attended a talk and press conference Barnard gave in London a couple of weeks after the event. He received a barrage of vitriolic criticism from members of the medical profession. He was accused of being an opportunistic interloper who had hijacked the opportunity after visiting the transplant researcher Norman Shumway in Stanford, California. 'He got there first because there were no regulatory authorities in South Africa' they said. Emboldened by post head injury disinhibition, I recall sticking my head above the parapet to exclaim 'no treatment that requires someone else to die first can ever prove mainstream' which is correct of course. American heart failure cardiologists described heart transplants as 'epidemiologically trivial' given the few donors and the plethora of severe heart failure patients less than sixty years of age.

Mr Donald Ross, a fellow South African who would become one of my mentors, was also at the presentation and within days performed Britain's first heart transplant at the National Heart Hospital. The circumstances surrounding the donor were controversial and the outcome a disaster but this was the case for many of the early attempts that followed Barnard's in the late 1960s. Others concurred about the paucity of donor hearts so baboon hearts were used opportunistically and Cambridge began a xenotransplantation research programme. But as Shumway would jest 'pig hearts are something for the future – and always will be!' So as long as humans provide the organs trauma and transplantation remain inextricably linked. The tests and strict criteria for defining brain death were put together specifically for the purpose of the transplant process. In countries like Japan where religious beliefs stipulate that

'SCOOP AND RUN' OR 'STAY AND PLAY'

the deceased's body must be maintained intact, surgeons were accused of murder for transplanting a heart.

For the 25th anniversary of Barnard's first transplant, the University of Cape Town put on a celebratory meeting for which I was invited to give a lecture on ventricular assist devices. This was the perfect opportunity to meet one of the world's surgical heroes. Barnard was heart surgeon turned cosmetics salesman by then but I liked him personally. Perhaps that was because we had stuff in common. A poor background. The need to make a difference. A difficult working environment and the uncomfortable drive to be first.

It was during that trip that I was asked to see an injured child in the Red Cross Children's Hospital. A gas canister had exploded in his township hovel and he suffered severe burns to his face and upper body, but critically to his windpipe which was largely destroyed and asphyxiating the boy. They knew I had designed an artificial windpipe so his doctors wondered whether I could use it to reconstruct the child's airways. Pressed for time on that occasion, I returned to Cape Town six weeks later and operated while supporting the lad on a heart-lung machine. Without needing to breathe or be ventilated, that gave me the exposure for an extensive reconstruction which changed his life. Having called in to see Barnard at Groote Schuur Hospital, I took the famous Blue Train to Johannesburg so I could visit the notorious Baragwaneth Hospital before flying home. The ticket was a gift in gratitude for my philanthropic journey to help the lad. Whatever it cost me it was a great privilege to do so.

Baragwaneth was infamous for the huge number of penetrating trauma victims brought in from the lawless townships. So much so that even one of its doctors was stabbed to death shortly before my arrival. It wasn't remotely similar to an American trauma centre, but they had sensible and effective ways of dealing with stab wounds to the chest. First, there was no tinkering pre-hospital care. ATLS didn't exist there. And unless the patient was exsanguinating from the heart or a major vessel, they just shoved in a chest drain, sucked out the blood, injected a dose of penicillin, then sent them out again. There was no exploratory surgery unless the blood kept coming down the tube. What's more, the patients seldom came back unless they were stabbed again. Contrast that with Britain, where virtually every patient would have a bucketful of fluid before a precautionary, exploratory operation then spend a week in hospital recovering from the painful incision rather than the original stab wound. It is what it is, but if I adopted the South African approach I would be sued in no time.

Sometime after the Cape Town meeting, I received a note from Barnard announcing that he had been asked to address the Oxford Union then give a talk at a Cambridge College the following evening. I invited him to watch some congenital heart surgery at the John Radcliffe Hospital and volunteered to drive him across country so as to avoid the convoluted rail journey via London. Something he was pleased to do. Since I was writing 'Landmarks' I wanted to hear the details of the first ever heart transplant from the horse's mouth. It was my opportunity to uncover the controversial details that others had missed.

Speeding out of Oxford in my blue Jaguar, I asked Barnard to discuss the thorny issues of apartheid and whether he would have been allowed to use a 'coloured' heart donor. Apparently that was off limits and the recipient, Louis Washkansky, almost died waiting as a result. By the time we drove into Cambridge through Trumpington I had learned more intrigue about his personal life than secrets surrounding the operation. I diverted past the Botanical Gardens towards St Mary's Convent school because I wanted young Gemma, my daughter, to meet the great man. An elderly nun, Sister Francesca, answered the door. She knew me well enough and was as excited as a nun can be to see that I had brought the famous Christiaan Barnard to say hello. More nuns came to the arched wooden porch, eager to cast eyes on the celebrity they had all heard about on the news. Then Gemma arrived and was happy to see her wayward dad, if only for five minutes. She politely shook Barnard's hand, kissed me goodbye then went back to her biology lesson about earthworms. That evening she told her mother 'Daddy turned up at school today with an old man. He was very tall and thin with long fingers but I didn't catch his name. The teachers seemed to know who he was.'

It was 1997 when I last heard from Barnard. He had just lost a friend in a tragic motor vehicle accident in Europe and wanted to talk. Why call me in Oxford? Perhaps because he knew I was producing a new book on thoracic trauma with Professor John O'Dell, his successor at Groote Schuur. Moreover, he knew that I had met the victim. Whatever the motive, he pressed me on whether she could have been saved. He thought so, and the whole debate was centred upon the 'stay and play' controversy. At the time I just listened to him and kept my opinions to myself. That said, the case made international headlines and was widely discussed in the media.

Some days later we took time to consider the circumstances in an educational forum in my department. I had encountered 'morbidity and mortality' meetings in the US then introduced them at the Hammersmith Hospital and Oxford. Poor outcomes were presented openly, blow by blow, so that deaths were learned from not swept under the carpet. Inevitably there was more to be gleaned from failure than the successes which were broadly expected from us.

This particular death occurred after a high speed road traffic accident involving abrupt deceleration and rotational forces. There were four people in the car, two of whom died at the scene. They were in Trunkey's early unsalvageable category. Not surprisingly, autopsy confirmed traumatic transection of the thoracic aorta with rapid exsanguination in both. Neither of them was wearing a seat belt. A third male passenger, restrained by a seat belt next to the driver, suffered severe head and facial injuries but survived.

The controversy arose in relation to the treatment of a young female in her mid-thirties seated behind the belted survivor. At the moment of impact, she was turned sideways facing her fellow rear seat passenger and was cushioned from being thrown through the windscreen.

Witnesses were soon on the scene including a passing doctor. He found the woman slumped uncomfortably in the rear well of the car and not easy to extricate from the wreckage. She was described as being conscious but dazed and groaning from a blow to the head. While breathing adequately she complained of pain in the right chest. I should explain at this point that the accident occurred in the centre of a large city and in proximity to teaching hospitals with both casualty and Thoracic Surgery departments.

In minutes, the site was cordoned off by a resuscitation-trained fire crew who needed to remove the car roof to free the occupants. The experienced sergeant in charge reported the victim as repeatedly crying 'oh my god, what's happened.' Then 'leave me alone,' as the reality of the situation impacted upon her. He had no difficulty in palpating a pulse at the wrist so, from our estimate, she had not lost a life-threatening quantity of blood at that point. The sergeant attempted to keep her calm and still during the extrication process and subsequently told the inquest 'I never thought she would die.'

It took thirty-five minutes to lift her from the wreckage, during which time an ambulance with a specialist emergency doctor had arrived. During the change in position, she suffered an abrupt loss of consciousness that was interpreted as a cardiac arrest. Presumably the attendants could not feel a pulse at that moment and they began external cardiac compressions. However there was no electrocardiographic confirmation of cardiac arrest and a defibrillator was not used. Pulses were detected when she was placed supine on the stretcher and she regained consciousness in the ambulance.

When doctors are dispatched to an accident with the remit to intervene that is precisely what they will do. Sitting in a control room all night doesn't cut it. 'Stay and play' becomes the order of the day. The ATLS protocols were followed assiduously in those days with two litres of clear fluid infused to raise the blood pressure. Thus, an intravenous cannula was inserted but by all accounts

THE TRAUMA CHRONICLES

the concussed and agitated patient pulled it straight out again.

As the clock ticked on the decision was taken to insert another cannula, inject sedative drugs then pass a tube in her windpipe to ventilate her. That would establish complete control but the consequences of those actions are predictable. Remember the Pennsylvania study that showed a fourfold increased risk of death for patients who underwent intubation before reaching hospital? The reason for that is straight forward as we have said. Sedation and paralysis blunt the body's response to its own adrenaline, causes a fall in blood pressure and significantly impairs cardiac contractility. To reiterate, positive pressure ventilation then raises the pressure within the chest, and slows the return of blood to the heart through the veins. In the presence of free blood or blood clot in the sac around the heart, those effects are further enhanced. And the pressure rises within the skull as a result. That's why all this is best done with careful monitoring in the hospital setting.

Clearly no one knew what the lady's internal injuries were. Two passengers were dead already and, in a high speed deceleration scenario, that was likely to be from ruptured aorta as the autopsies confirmed. Consideration should have been given to the fact that the third unrestrained passenger had life-threatening internal injuries too. In my view, that likelihood itself dictates the need for 'scoop and run' so the correct diagnosis can be made and surgery undertaken rapidly. Needless to say, Champion was in full agreement with that, but those on site were only following guidelines. The interventions were considered in the patient's best interest in their system at that time.

184

'SCOOP AND RUN' OR 'STAY AND PLAY'

Whatever the circumstances in the back of that ambulance, it didn't leave the crash site for seventy-seven minutes after the time of impact, a full forty-two minutes after the victim was released from the wreckage. It then took another twenty-five minutes to reach the hospital four miles away so the critical 'Golden Hour' had long expired.

What happened after the drugs and intubation? Predictably, the blood pressure dropped away requiring large volumes of clear fluid and cardiac stimulant drugs. The ambulance actually had to pull over and stop en route to enable the resuscitation efforts.

More than an hour and a half from the time of the crash she was delivered into the hands of hospital doctors, but there was no senior surgeon present. By then, her pulses were no longer palpable and the body temperature had fallen with high levels of acid in the bloodstream. Fearful of losing her, a chest X-ray was taken within minutes of arrival. This reportedly showed fractured ribs on the right side and some blood around the lung.

So parlous was the poor woman's condition now that the emergency room doctors urged an on call surgery resident to open her chest right there in the reception area. Unfortunately, the trainee didn't find significant bleeding to stop. In the meantime, an experienced cardiac surgeon arrived but by the time he joined the operation the situation was grave. He elected to extend the incision across the breastbone and into the left side where he began open chest cardiac massage.

What injuries did he find? That was the question I put to the Morbidity and Mortality meeting. I already knew the details from Barnard who had described the autopsy findings to me.

THE TRAUMA CHRONICLES

I asked the juniors what the possibilities were, knowing full well that they wouldn't get it.

'Put yourself in the position of the pre-hospital team,' I said. 'What were they likely to be treating? Was it a good move to pass the tracheal tube and ventilate the woman at the crash site?'

'Not just to keep her quiet,' chirped one feisty student.

'It was intended to facilitate the vein cannulation,' I responded defensively. One of the junior registrars chipped in with 'it was a high speed injury so maybe she had a torn aorta or bronchus.'

'Think about that,' I said. 'If the bleeding came from the aorta she'd have died much sooner. And if a bronchus was ruptured her head and neck would have blown up like a balloon when they ventilated her.'

The savvy senior registrar considered blunt cardiac trauma, perhaps with a leaking heart valve, as the likely explanation for the blood pressure changes. That could have happened had the chest impacted against the head rest of the front seat.

Moreover, the aggressive fluid infusion would have worsened heart failure under those conditions which fitted the clinical picture.

One by one we worked through the possibilities, but the real answer didn't come. I was not surprised. The 'mechanism of injury,' as we call it, was unusual for the seat belt era. Deceleration and torsion through twisting to the right best described it. The chest can be viewed as a bell shaped structure with the heavy blood-containing structures in the middle like the clanger. What deceleration impact does is to bring the bell itself to an abrupt standstill while the momentum of the clanger keeps it swinging. The heavy column of blood that is the aorta then tears where it is fixed to the spine at the back by its branches.

The heart is heavy, too, but is normally cushioned by the breast bone in front and the spine behind. However, if the blow impacts from the side the heart will twist on its axis to produce a torsion injury. With a hefty blow, a torn or burst pericardial sac is well described. So what did the senior surgeon find?

As he urgently began the internal cardiac compressions he discovered a tear in the fibrous sac that 'he could put his fist through.' But pericardial lacerations don't bleed significantly, so where had the blood come from? It was not that easy to find the hole in the upper of the two veins draining into the heart from the left lung. It was tucked away behind the ventricles at the back of the chest but, that said, it was a simple job to close the rent with a couple of stitches.

As Barnard himself wrote about the incident, 'the injury that caused the bleeding was a vein which didn't bleed quickly, in fact it bleeds rather slowly.' A woman's superior pulmonary vein is around 1.5 cms in diameter and 3 cms in length. The pressure within it is no more than 15mm Hg compared to more than 120mm Hg in an artery. Blood clot covering the tear would normally prove sufficient to stop the haemorrhage as the pressure within the veins fell.

Despite the best efforts of an experienced cardiac surgeon, the metabolic derangement made it impossible to revive her. So many vials of adrenalin were used in fruitless attempts to restart the heart that the hospital ran out. At the inquest, the pathologist stated 'the injury was small, but in the wrong place. If she had worn a seatbelt she would have been fine.' Sad but true. Some believe that she could have survived without any treatment at all.

From my own perspective, the description of a sudden loss of blood pressure during extrication from the vehicle was compatible with the position change displacing the ventricles through the torn sac. If not, the cardiac compressions would have done so, and it's obvious that only surgery can close holes in a blood vessel. Pouring in fluid to raise the blood pressure cannot help so we're back to the leaking vessel analogy. A hole halfway up a plastic bottle of orange squash will leak, and the more water you pour in, the more diluted the orange becomes. It's the same with haemoglobin and clotting factors in the blood. To continuously dilute the circulation with clear fluid reduces both the oxygen carrying capacity and metabolic function so the poor heart can't function. So is it better to 'scoop and run' and avoid pre-hospital resuscitation? My own experience certainly suggests that.

One weekend when I was a senior registrar on call in the Middlesex Hospital, I was alerted to the arrival of an ambulance bringing in a teenager who had been shot in the left chest by the police in a stake out. The lad arrived in the accident department just behind Oxford Street half an hour after the incident. As for the patient in question he was awake, anxious and in shock with a blood pressure of 85 mm Hg. Blue distended jugular veins stood out in his neck against pale, sweaty skin. Thankfully it was 1985 so he had received no efforts at pre-hospital resuscitation. I rested my fingers on the faint pulse at the wrist and briskly walked with the stretcher to the X-ray

'SCOOP AND RUN' OR 'STAY AND PLAY'

department. Meanwhile the operating theatres were warned to make ready for us.

The X-ray showed what I anticipated. The wide heart shadow suggested a collection of blood clot in the pericardial sac and there was free blood in both chest cavities. The spent low velocity bullet was in the right chest just above the diaphragm and the position of the entry wound made me certain that it had passed directly through the heart and both lungs. We arrived in theatre without any drips or fluids and he was quickly put to sleep by an anaesthetic trainee who was also on call in the hospital. Predictably, the blood pressure dropped when the anaesthetic drugs were injected and the windpipe tubed. But we were prepared and ready with bags of uncross-matched blood and two large cannulas in place to counter the deterioration.

As his blood pressure disappeared I opened him quickly, straight up the breastbone then through the front of the pericardial sac and scooped out the clots. The relief of cardiac tamponade caused the pressure to rise spontaneously. What's more, there was surprisingly little bleeding from the separate holes in his right and left atria, the two low pressure chambers of the heart. They were plugged by sticky blood clot which obscured them and were easily closed with a couple of nylon stitches. By way of analogy, this lad had a double dose of the unfortunate woman in the car accident. Same sized holes in low pressure chambers. He left the hospital five days later, sore, angry, but unscathed. Rescued by a trainee surgeon.

Years later in Oxford, I was called at night about a shocked patient with a high velocity rifle wound through the left chest. Shot mistakenly by a poacher, he had been retrieved from a rural site, taken to the nearest general

THE TRAUMA CHRONICLES

hospital but passed on like a hot potato without any intervention at all. Absence of delay saved his life. The man had already lost two litres of blood into the left chest cavity so it was already forty to love on our bleeding scale.

I arrived in the Emergency room before the ambulance and had an anaesthetist waiting. I simply opened him right there on the trolley and put a clamp across the hilum of the lung before we transfused him with blood. The bullet had passed straight through the main artery which bleeds profusely until the pressure within it falls. But he had still reached hospital alive an hour after the event. Once we had rendered him stable, I took him to the operating theatre to remove the lung and he also recovered uneventfully.

Clearly I have sympathy for those doing their best in difficult circumstances in accordance with their guidelines, but informed trauma care is about predicting the worst case scenario and accommodating it. It needs diagnosis focused intervention not knee jerk reactions to altered vital signs irrespective of the risks.

The contemporary thinking on pre-hospital care was summarised recently in an article published in the American Journal of Emergency Medical Services. It was written by experienced emergency technicians that have to do the job. 'One of the most critical pre-hospital treatment interventions for trauma patients is to limit scene time. Every minute that pre-hospital providers spend on trauma scenes increases patient mortality.' Hence the clear message is scoop and run unless there is a compelling reason not to.

On Saturday 2nd September, 2001, in Paphos, Cyprus, the charismatic Christiaan Barnard suffered a severe asthmatic attack in a swimming pool. He grappled for an inhaler but collapsed and died a lonely man far from home. Remembered by some for all the wrong reasons. When asked by the BBC to make a programme to commemorate the 50th anniversary of the first heart transplant, I did my best to give the man the credit he rightly deserved. I located all the surviving members of the operating team on that memorable night and they all spoke highly of him. His charming daughter Deirdre told me 'the world took dad away from us for a while, but eventually he came back.' I know just what she meant.

GETTING THERE

If you want the rainbow, you gotta put up
with rain

Dolly Parton

Improvements in care for the injured eventually emerged through the dedication and enthusiasm of individuals who sought change in their own hospitals and regions. Some of those surgeons were with us on Miles Irving's Royal College of Surgeons Committee in 1988, though sadly the influence of our 'unnecessary deaths' study was temporary at best.

When I left London for Oxford in 1986, the accident statistics for the new M25 motorway were a major cause for concern. From Harefield, I had covered a quarter of the circumference of that orbital road with numerous urgent visits to general hospitals both within and outside its perimeter. Great experience for me, hit or miss for the patients since it took between minutes and days for me to reach them.

That same year, the affable Accident and Emergency Specialist, Dr Alistair Wilson, of the Royal London Hospital, wrote a pointed letter to the Assistant Commissioner of Police at New Scotland Yard. The crux of his message was as follows, 'At the moment, people are dying because we are unable to provide sufficient expertise at the accident site. This mortality is exaggerated when the current slow road transport of victims, often without adequate ongoing resuscitation, is added.' Of course the Royal London was destined to become a major trauma centre and leading light in specialty, but it is curious how serendipity rather than politics can play a key role in such developments.

The following year, Wilson wrote another letter:

There is currently carnage daily on the M25 which is not being serviced properly and that, unless people use helicopters which are appropriately medically staffed and equipped, the carnage is likely to get much worse. In particular, there is nobody in this country properly trained, it strikes me, in disaster techniques.

Of course, many of us knew that the US trauma centres were using helicopter retrieval manned by medics on a routine basis. As revealed by the archives of the London Air Ambulance Service, it was a chance conversation on a tennis court that kicked off the UK initiative. The wife of the Royal London surgeon, Richard Earlam, was in conversation with Lady Stevens of Ludgate, wife of the Chairman of United Newspapers plc. Curiously, they happened to be discussing the superiority of trauma care in Germany and, by chance, formed the basis for a charity partnership that would fund London's first rescue helicopter. Needless to say the caring NHS wasn't about to chip in. Ultimately that was a mistake in my view. Highlighting the hideous number of unnecessary trauma deaths helped at that point. It was predicted that improved pre-hospital care could save around 200 lives per year in the Metropolitan region.

The *Express* newspaper group agreed to contribute £4 million to fund the first helicopter with pilots, operational staff and running costs for four years—an initiative that gained support from Margaret Thatcher and her government. Surprisingly, soon after that in December 1988, the French-built Aerospatiale SA 365N arrived and the Helicopter Emergency Medical Service was born. Needless to say it was continued on a charitable basis, and the first mission was not on behalf of an injured patient but on an organ donor run from Scotland to London. As we have said, organ donation is an important side-line in the trauma world, but the success of the two are inversely related. The more patients who die through inadequate care, the more organs are available for transplant. That's life, or perhaps death.

By 1990, the rescue helicopter carried both a doctor and a London ambulance service paramedic and, given the ongoing need for independent financial support, the service was widely publicised. Unfortunately not always in a credible fashion. In June that year the *Times* showed a photograph of the helicopter which had landed in Hammersmith. The caption 'Street incredibility: Bemused residents stare at the helicopter ambulance that landed with a patient in Fulham Palace Road outside Charing Cross Hospital, London yesterday.' One has to ask why, and of course many did.

On another occasion, when a young man was mauled by a lion in London Zoo, one of Britain's major teaching centres, University College Hospital, was less than a mile away. But the helicopter arrived spectacularly at great expense and carried the patient off to the London Hospital. The spat between the two was played out in the public eye, and similar contentious episodes followed. It all served to keep trauma on the agenda, but when a service is funded by the media, it is particularly difficult to hide from it.

Given that broken bones are encountered much more frequently than shattered organs in most Accident Departments, it was the British Orthopaedic Association who endeavoured to gain improvements. Their detailed review of NHS trauma services illustrated in stark fashion that treatment of the injured lagged woefully behind the advances made in the rest of Europe. That's when things began to change in Oxford.

The Chief Executive of our hospitals at the time was Nigel Crisp, a Cambridge educated philosophy graduate, now Lord Crisp, who went on to run London's healthcare then the whole of the NHS. Nigel had already overseen the huge and controversial advances in my own department. One morning in 1993, two innovative young orthopaedic surgeons, Keith Willett and Peter Worlock, knocked on his door and asked for support in designing an improved trauma service for the expansive Oxford Region. They argued that given the vital 'Golden Hour,' it was essential to have a trauma surgeon in the hospital around the clock. That was the only way to have sufficient expertise on site for every single patient. But they knew that it was destined to prove controversial.

Willett's strategy had been carefully planned over many months. As Crisp put it, 'It was a Chief Executive's dream; a fully thought out proposal which improved quality without additional cost. They had foreseen how other roles would have to change, with nurses taking on tasks previously reserved for doctors.' We had already set that precedent in cardiac surgery where advanced nurse practitioners were responsible for post-operative care and mobilising patients through our fast track cardiac recovery unit. And after tremendous rows with both the Royal Colleges of Surgeons and Nursing, I had introduced US-style surgical nurse practitioners in my operating theatres to dissect out the leg veins for coronary bypass surgery. They did it better than trainee surgeons. So Oxford was used to rocking the boat.

Willett and Worlock trained their own advanced nurse practitioners to manage injured patients, alongside the new role of 'trauma technician' to take over a variety of roles from doctors and nurses. They even established a research programme to examine the effects of the new hospital rotas on surgeons and their families and the overall effects on patient care. As one might expect the establishment hated the prospect of consultant surgeons being resident and working in the hospital overnight. They feared it would become a bridgehead from which management could insist that all consultants should be available around the clock. And just as they had responded negatively to our cardiac initiatives, they resented the expanded roles and responsibility of the nurses. It was a misguided, self-interested and even pathetic response that ignored the fact that nurses had 'ruled the roost' in traditional Casualty Departments for many years.

As Sister in Charge of the Accident Departments in Cambridge, then the Royal Free and St Thomas' Hospital in London, my own wife, Sarah, had invariably taken responsibility for organising appropriate treatment for the injured. What else could senior nurses do when inexperienced trainee doctors were the only medical staff available for dire emergencies, especially at night?

THE TRAUMA CHRONICLES

Dithering doesn't do it. Sister was 'queen bee.' When Sarah called for help the surgeons came running – if only to spend some time with her.

As Lord Crisp reminisced, 'I remember how the Royal College of Surgeons representative on the interview panel actually tried to put candidates off the three new consultant posts that were needed. He failed. The bright young surgeons we appointed in 1994 were incredibly enthusiastic to be part of this visionary service which they regarded as being the way for the future.'

Perhaps that vexatious, self-interested attitude of the day explained why the college's Trauma Committee recommendations five years previously had failed to make headway. But there was a revolution happening in Oxford. Trauma orthopaedic operations were separated from elective surgery, and when the brain surgeons relocated to Oxford's main hospital we had everything we needed for a front line trauma centre. That included a helicopter landing pad already used for transplant donor runs. Yet that wasn't the point, really. As Ross Davenport from the London Hospital put it 'Trauma centres needed to be specialist hospitals, not just hospitals with specialties.'

The NHS is such a centralised political organisation that nothing changes without moving mountains. Of course it helped to have surgeons in a position of political influence, and that happened with the appointment of the Professor of Surgery of St Mary's Hospital to a Ministerial post. Lord Ara Darzi's review of healthcare in London in 2007 confirmed the widely debated deficiencies in the treatment of the injured and the unnecessary loss of life that ensued. Given that trauma care had been repeatedly shown to be unsatisfactory the

GETTING THERE

antiquated system really had to be reformed, just as we had emphasised twenty years before.

Darzi formally recommended that a 'hub and spoke' trauma system should be established for the capital so that patients with serious injuries could be conveyed directly to one of a small number of major trauma centres. So at last the edict went out. Split London into four segments with a specialised trauma centre in each. The hospitals chosen were Darzi's own St Mary's Hospital in the north west segment, the Royal London in the north east, then correspondingly St George's and King's College Hospitals south of the river.

Lord Darzi went on to write a report about the whole country and, not surprisingly, Oxford became the next designated trauma centre. We already functioned as such. It was the era of appointing National Clinical Directors, or Tsars as they were called, for specialities such as cancer or diabetes, and it seemed obvious that the formal reorganisation of trauma care should have one too. Who better than Keith Willett with his proven expertise in the area?

Willett became National Clinical Director for Trauma Care in 2009 with the specific remit to implement regional networks for care of the injured throughout the NHS. It was a timely appointment given that a National Audit Office report the following year showed Oxford to be the only hospital to provide round the clock specialist cover, and in the rest of the country a staggering 64% of major trauma patients still never received senior medical input.

At this stage, the designated major trauma centres would serve around three to four million people each, and be equipped and staffed to manage major injuries on

· 199

a round the clock basis. In turn, the pre-hospital services were provided with protocols to ensure that their patients reached an appropriate hospital for their condition in an acceptable time frame. In Oxford, there was a consultant resuscitation team leader in the Emergency Department at all times supported by senior nurses. There had to be round the clock access to x-rays and a CT scanner together with constant laboratory and blood bank support. Specialist orthopaedic, neurosurgical, plastic, vascular and cardiothoracic surgeons were all on call at short notice alongside specialist anaesthetists. The surgeons were expected to attend an ATLS course, while a new Pre-Hospital Life Support course was established for paramedics.

A four step triage algorithm was devised based on the patient's vital signs: the anatomical location of the injury, the circumstances of the accident and then any other contributing factors that might influence the decision as to those who should be taken directly to a trauma centre. Primarily all unconscious patients, and those in shock with a blood pressure less than 90 mm Hg, were to be taken there directly. Next, those with a significant chest injury, traumatic amputation of a limb, penetrating wound to the neck, chest or abdomen, and those with fractures of the skull, pelvis or spine should follow the same route. A third group were patients with a notably high risk mechanism of injury such as rapid deceleration where others have died, or a fall from greater than 20 feet. The last consideration was for injured patients with complex circumstances including pregnancy, morbid obesity, or a bleeding disorder who served to benefit from a high degree of expertise.

GETTING THERE

Given the degree of urgency for these groups, an acceptable transport time was thought to be in the order of thirty to forty-five minutes. While it took time to become comfortable with driving past the front door of a nearby general hospital this had to be the right thing given the sad state of affairs beforehand. Within months the better staffed and equipped trauma centres were shown to reduce the incidence of preventable deaths. Ambulance transport times throughout the London network were modest, with 93% of patients arriving within 30 minutes and 74% within 20 minutes. And most were still treated on a 'scoop and run' basis at that stage.

Against this background, the controversy over the role of helicopters raged on in the public eye. Given my experiences in the US, I had been a firm advocate of helicopter retrieval during that Royal College of Surgeons Working Party. But I envisaged its role under NHS direction for long distance retrieval from motorways or remote rural locations where road ambulance transport times were likely to prove excessive. Inner city use was questionable as was competition between charitable providers. Were disruptive helicopter landings in the middle of the city of London an advisable option to begin such an initiative?

Then, on 24 April 1993, a truck bomb was detonated in Bishopsgate. One passer-by was killed outright and forty-four others injured. The air ambulance arrived, with an independent television film crew in tow. It was 'show biz' medicine and surgery played out on the streets for the cameras without any of the confidentiality normally afforded to the sick. There were several teaching hospital Accident Departments close by which raised the question as to whether pre-hospital care was needed or indeed ethical. The bombers made their point for the anti-air ambulance lobby.

Next came 'successful open heart surgery at the roadside' on Christmas Eve, 1993, outside the Kismet Indian Restaurant. As the air ambulance charity put it on their advertising literature:

The world's first successful open heart surgery at the roadside challenged the guidelines on resuscitation. The non-conventional approach and personal courage of individual doctors pushed the boundaries of pre-hospital care and continues to save lives today.

Really? I certainly applauded that effort. Any life saved by decisive intervention should be celebrated, but a certain Ludwig Rehn of Frankfurt had done the same in September 1896 and surgeons have performed out of hospital thoracotomy for penetrating wounds ever since. Doing it in the road for a curry house audience was hardly a great medical advance. And the way that it was publicised caused disdain. Sad to say that many contemporary television programmes about pre-hospital care prove cringeworthy too, however well intentioned.

By 1994, the Department of Health decided to take a careful look at the performance of the London Air Ambulance Service and, of course, anecdote and objective analysis often tell a different story. What became known as the Sheffield Report concluded that there was no evidence for improved survival or improved health outcomes for air ambulance patients. Critics said the money would be better spent elsewhere but the 'star struck' general public were angered and supportive. It was the perfect opportunity for Richard Branson and the Virgin Group to arrive on a white charger, purchase the helicopter and paint it red with the Virgin logo on the side. Richard said 'I realised it was time to pay back,' having been rescued five times by helicopter himself during his adventures abroad. All donations were tax deductible.

Perhaps the most significant contribution came when rapid response cars were introduced for night operations. When the dreadful Paddington train crash happened on 5 October 1999, the single helicopter was out of action for mechanical repairs. On that occasion, the Air Ambulance Service delivered four advanced trauma teams by road to the railway station and helped to coordinate the triage response alongside the conventional ambulance service. Sadly, thirty-one people died and 220 were injured. The splendid St Mary's Hospital, one hundred yards away from the tracks, took the brunt of that event and was backed up by the Hammersmith, Westminster & Chelsea and other first class acute hospitals in the vicinity.

What do advanced trauma teams actually do in the pre-hospital setting? As in the French system it began with putting cannulas into veins and pouring in clear fluid. Then they progressed to the insertion of breathing tubes into the windpipe. As we have said, both can be lifesaving procedures but both can cause harm too. By the time our pre-hospital responders had started to administer intravenous fluids the Americans were warning against it.

I have emphasised that it is not possible to gauge the amount of bleeding a patient has suffered by measuring vital signs by the roadside. In the real world, human physiology doesn't respond in a reproducible manner in a set time frame. For instance a slow heart rate can be found during major haemorrhage. Why? One theory is that the body mounts a two phase response to bleeding. In the beginning, an outpouring of adrenaline with fright causes rapid heart rate and elevated blood pressure through constriction of the small blood vessels. This is followed by a slower rate probably induced by the vagus nerve which controls the workings of our heart, lungs and guts. A theory to explain this is that bleeding into the abdomen around the viscera is responsible. Yet whatever the reason, all may not be as it seems. Raised pressure within the skull, various medications and the blunted physiological responses of the elderly may all play a part in the confusion.

In 1994, a US Consensus Panel on Resuscitation in Haemorrhagic Shock reported both patient and experimental evidence demonstrating improved survival when fluids were limited or withheld altogether until bleeding had been stopped surgically. And while ventilating through a tracheal tube may protect the unconscious, it can cause havoc for traumatised lungs should air leak into the chest cavity. The positive pressure worsens the leak causing air to build up under tension. Moreover, the mid-line structures, including the heart, can be pushed across into the opposite side of the chest to compress the uninjured lung. This is called tension pneumothorax and requires expedite relief by inserting a chest drain.

Pre-hospital doctors and advanced level paramedics are taught how to decompress a pneumothorax by inserting a needle through the chest wall between the ribs. Simple you might think but not as easy as it sounds particularly in the obese. Moreover a number of US investigations have shown the incidence of traumatic pneumothorax to be grossly exaggerated by pre-hospital responders. In one report there were twenty probing needle insertions for every tension pneumothorax found. Even after stab and gunshot wounds, the prevalence was as low as 0.3% in those who remained conscious when examined for breath sounds. Another paper reported that 60% of tension pneumothoraxes occurred simply because pre-hospital positive pressure ventilation caused thin-walled cysts on the lung surface to burst.

The next step was to teach out of hospital chest drain insertion which is something even I wouldn't wish to do without scrutinising a chest X-ray first. I've written about the dangers of that before in *The Knife's Edge*. Blindly inserted drains can penetrate both heart and lungs. Some end up in the abdominal cavity having traversed the diaphragm. Ultimately, the helicopter medics even decided they should open the chest in the street for suspected stab wounds to the heart. It was all laid out in those Advanced Trauma Life Support guidelines and enthusiastically advocated by the colourful vascular surgeon Karim Brohi, who worked as a helicopter medic in London.

Brohi set up a 'do it yourself' website called Trauma. org which promoted emergency chest opening as follows – 'Accepted indications include penetrating thoracic injury with unresponsive low blood pressure, less than 70 mm Hg, which the Americans wouldn't even transfuse for, or witnessed cardiac arrest, or blunt chest injury with unresponsive low blood pressure, or rapid bleeding (greater than 1,500 ml) from the chest tube.' So here's the scalpel; off you go! Just make sure you can handle what you find inside. Carving through the chest wall is the easy bit.

While I have opened a number of chests successfully in the Emergency Department I personally never did see a survivor from out of hospital thoracotomy. Sadly my team have even been called to close the chest up again after nothing of significance was found and the person who opened it didn't know what to do next. Uninspiring. In 2003, the American College of Surgeons noted 'although the United Kingdom, Germany, Spain and Japan have advocated pre-hospital thoracotomy for traumatic cardiac arrest, this is not a procedure we expect to be performed by paramedics.' I would add to that 'non-surgeons.' Most charitably-funded helicopters and emergency response vehicles are staffed by volunteers and enthusiasts of varied disciplines and levels of training. In Oxford, some are general practitioners but not Accident and Emergency doctors or surgeons.

When taught, and given free rein to perform a procedure, it is natural to want to get on and use it. I felt that way about drilling holes in the head, but there are risks attached to every procedure.

Nevertheless, credit where credit is due. The London Helicopter Emergency Services led the way with this aggressive approach and any life saved from the Grim Reaper's scythe is a bonus. A retrospective review of penetrating trauma patients with cardiac arrest between 1993 and 1999 reported thirty-nine pre-hospital thoracotomies performed with four patients surviving to hospital discharge. Three ostensibly had no brain damage while one was severely disabled.

While developments in London set the ball rolling, our prerogative was to roll out a trauma centre network across the whole country, and for that a national advisory group was assembled. This included medical experts from the relevant surgical specialties together with nurses, NHS managers and allied healthcare professionals. At last we had the basis for a patient-focused approach to major injuries encapsulating pre-hospital care, resuscitation and early surgery, and even including that 'Cinderella' of trauma care, rehabilitation. Strong directives were made and each region adapted them for their own geography and the population they served. At last, the priority was to get the injured patient to the right place at the right time for the right care.

The London hospitals covered a relatively small geographical area with short transport times by ambulance to one of the four major centres. Not so out in the countryside and in other cities where only one teaching hospital could provide the multiple specialist surgeons required to staff a trauma centre. For that reason, a three tiered system was adopted by designating some hospitals as major trauma centres, and others as secondary trauma units if the main centre couldn't be reached within 45 minutes. The remainder were categorised as local emergency hospitals catering for minor injuries. Specialist paediatric trauma units were established in twelve regional teaching hospitals alongside the four dedicated children's hospitals in Birmingham, Liverpool, Manchester and Sheffield.

In the absence of a countrywide air ambulance service, it was decided that severely injured patients with predictably long transfer times should first be taken to the nearest secondary trauma unit for resuscitation and control of life-threatening bleeding. All general hospitals have orthopaedic and abdominal surgeons, but head and chest injuries would only receive specialist care when transferred on to the major trauma centre. Paramedics called to the site of an incident took responsibility for deciding who should go where based upon an injury scoring system. Usually that worked out well, sometimes it didn't. Initial findings can prove deceptive and it is impossible to see into the body cavities.

By 2012, the 60 million population in the UK was covered by twenty-six major trauma centres who treated 16,000 patients between them. Twelve thousand of these were conveyed there directly. Others needing specialist surgery were referred on from a secondary trauma unit. On the positive side, the numbers receiving immediate attention from a consultant-led resuscitation team increased from 50% in 2011 to 75% in 2013. For unconscious patients, the proportion receiving a tracheal tube and artificial ventilation increased by the same percentage and 45% of diagnostic CT scans happened within 30 minutes of arrival to hospital. In particular 90% of patients with a head injury were scanned within an hour. Collectively this resulted in a one fifth reduction in deaths following injury throughout the country.

Happily, we were getting somewhere at last. So called 'damage control' resuscitation then evolved from the US to combat excessive clear fluid administration. So called 'permissive' low blood pressure became acceptable in trauma patients in order to avoid the lethal triad of clotting disturbances, hypothermia and metabolic derangement caused by the original ATLS guidelines. To pour in fluids as soon as possible was never the right thing. It was well intentioned but naïve. Like mechanical ventilation for Covid-19 patients, it damaged more patients than it saved. So 'permissive hypotension' simply aimed to

GETTING THERE

maintain a pre-surgery blood pressure averaging 65 mm Hg, just enough for a palpable pulse at the wrist and the same as my cardiac patients on the bypass machine. Should fluids be required for lower pressure they should be blood based products to maintain clotting, not clear fluids to destroy it. Simple. You don't need to be a doctor or paramedic to understand that.

By 2010 I had achieved the world's longest survivor by far with any type of artificial heart using a high speed rotary blood pump that rendered my patients pulseless. Literally pulseless because the high speed impeller produced continuous blood flow. It didn't empty and fill as the human heart does, or as the pulsatile total artificial hearts and left ventricular assist devices used to. My patients with these machines lived with a pressure within the blood stream between 80 mm Hg and 90 mm Hg. It came as a surprise to many that their brains and other organs worked fine with that physiology. So the target of restoring pulsatile blood pressure to levels greater than 100 mm Hg in trauma patients was never valid and innumerable patient's suffered because of that obsession.

An article from the US Journal 'Critical Care' made the following statement in 2008:

Evidence suggests no benefit with any single pre-hospital intervention. Furthermore data on pre-hospital intubation suggests the potential for harm particularly amongst patients with head injuries. Amongst those without head injuries who require immediate haemorrhage control, tracheal intubation is even less likely to be of benefit. The hospital procedures needed to affect outcome in the

THE TRAUMA CHRONICLES

bleeding patient are simply delayed by interventions performed in the pre-hospital setting.

That was clear enough. Now consider this curious and recent case from the streets of London. A team of two NHS paramedics in an ambulance were called to a young man who had been shot in the neck by a hand gun. They arrived to find the distressed patient lying on the pavement but fully conscious, breathing without difficulty and with raised blood pressure through sheer agitation and distress. He recalled the incident in detail stating that a man on a moped had pulled up alongside him, taken the pistol from a jacket pocket, then shot him at point blank range. Sure enough the paramedics found a single bullet entry wound in the left side of the man's throat which they judged to be close to the windpipe. Fortunately, despite the major blood vessels in the neck being very close to the wound, there was no significant bleeding. Lucky man. Obviously it was a low velocity bullet, and in the absence of an exit wound it remained in his neck. When consigned to the job the NHS paramedics were told to inform the separate Helicopter Emergency Medical Services about the patient's status. Then they would decide whether the case warranted their attention. From then onwards the tale becomes progressively more bizarre.

Over the radio the paramedics straightforwardly explained their findings and their plan to 'blue light' the victim to the nearest major trauma centre some three miles away, a five minute drive. Given that the man complained of numbness in his left hand they suggested stabilising his head and neck with an external collar in case the bullet was causing pressure on the spinal cord

210

GETTING THERE

or nerve plexus supplying the arm. At that point, the remote and uninformed advice was not to support the neck as the airway and breathing took priority. So, still breathing and talking normally, the man walked into the back of the ambulance where the paramedics rechecked the pulse rate, blood pressure and oxygen saturation all of which remained completely normal. Still the only complaint was of altered sensation in the left hand because the foreign body was compressing a nerve root.

I would add at this point that one of the paramedics is a young man whom I greatly respect. He was at school with my son then a soldier who served during conflict in the Middle East, dodging bullets himself and rescuing his wounded colleagues. That's why he decided to become a paramedic in civilian life. With the trauma centre expecting the patient within minutes the ambulance set off. But they didn't get far. They were radioed by the control room and told to pull over until an Emergency Medical Services doctor and paramedic could reach them by car to assess the patient. Curious, because there were hospitals full of doctors close by so why put one out on the road? They clearly didn't trust the paramedics.

Of course their findings were just the same—steady pulse, good blood pressure, normal oxygen levels in a fully conscious patient who could tell the story. The interlopers then made two botched attempts to insert a cannula into a vein and set up a drip that the patient clearly didn't need. Having failed miserably in that endeavour the ambulance was allowed to proceed to the hospital with the doctor's car following behind. One doctor and three paramedics with a walking wounded patient.

THE TRAUMA CHRONICLES

From my own standpoint, I regard that as wholly inexplicable interference with the patient's treatment pathway. How did the NHS come to accept that from a charity? My paramedic friend was neither complaining nor telling tales out of school. I had simply asked him whether he had seen any interesting cases since his last visit, then probed him on a story that seemed so bizarre. He's a young man who is keen to learn and often asks me what I would do in difficult situations. Yet it seems that competition between pre-hospital care groups is a recurring theme. Paramedics report that, having arrived at an accident, they are instructed to linger at the scene waiting for a helicopter to arrive rather than conveying their patient to hospital—it is a source of frustration and something the injured could well do without. So how does the system work?

It costs around £10.5 million each year to run the London Helicopter Emergency Medical Service which dispatches a doctor and a paramedic to the scene of an accident or life-threatening medical event such as a cardiac arrest. But remember it takes time to organise a flight and arrange to land on city roads. Dying people can't wait for that. That considerable sum is accumulated from charitable donations with 53 pence per pound paying for the fund raising efforts leaving less than half for service provision. The stated remit of the Service is to 'blend a combination of civilian medical care with aspects of aviation and military practice' to provide intensive trauma care to people with life-threatening problems at the site. It's the stay and play role, while the NHS ambulance service predominantly provides scoop and run. And that includes performing surgery in the street.

212

GETTING THERE

How do they find their patients? A London air ambulance paramedic sits in the NHS Ambulance Service control room monitoring and interrogating more than 4,500 999 calls per day, sifting for the type of patient who might theoretically benefit from a trauma team response. In the meantime, an 'experienced trauma team doctor' and an advanced paramedic sit waiting to intervene for what averages out at five patients per day. It's not surprising, then, that when dispatched they insist upon doing something. There are now twenty independent regional air ambulance organisations using a total of thirty-seven helicopters, each operating on similar principles and competing with each other for work.

Getting the injured into an operating theatre with the right surgeon is what matters most. As one eminent Accident and Emergency doctor put it 'helicopters are not therapy, merely transport.' And a number of studies have highlighted the fact that air transport does not expedite hospital admission unless the accident is more than 45 kilometres away. There are reasons for this. Urban areas virtually always have a conventional ambulance station with paramedics in proximity while there is inherent delay for logistical planning before a helicopter can be dispatched to the chosen landing site. A review published in a surgical journal showed that the discontinuation of a regional helicopter air ambulance service did not negatively influence any aspect of trauma mortality and actually shortened transport times. Another detailed analysis presented in the Annals of the Royal College of Surgeons examined the spectrum of injured patients brought into a single hospital over a 20 month period by the Oxfordshire, Wiltshire and

Berkshire Air Ambulances. Of the 111 cases with sufficient data to be included, forty-five were classified as walking wounded with minor injuries and discharged home from the accident department. Only twenty-four needed any form of surgery, ten of which were admitted to intensive care afterwards. Given that helicopter retrieval costs at least £6000 per event and was meant to address the seriously injured, the surgeon authors were scathing about the management of emergency services who appeared unable to make sensible triage decisions.

Having been a firm advocate for the introduction of helicopter retrieval on that first College of Surgeons Trauma Committee, I still believe the service has an important role, particularly in rural areas when addressing the 'Golden Hour' trauma deaths that are critically time dependant. But the system should have been part of the NHS, not run by disparate charities. And ultimately it's the statistics that matter, not anecdotes. That said, the efforts of the doctors and paramedics on board are greatly appreciated by those that they rescue and the general public. I just don't think that the media helps by intruding nor glorifying routine and simple procedures just because they are undertaken outside the hospital environment.

Should this read as if I am against pre-hospital care the opposite is true. I was and still am working on a new portable circulatory support system to rescue victims of out of hospital cardiac arrest and enable transport of the desperately sick from a general hospital to a cardiac centre. But wherever possible, resuscitation efforts must take place with the diagnosis in mind and in a controlled environment supported by the right staff, drugs and equipment. Only a hospital provides that.

To Mend a Broken Heart

Yesterday I was clever so I wanted to change the
world. Today I am wise so I am changing myself.

Rumi

Of the hundreds of patients I've treated with chest
injuries throughout the world, relatively few actually
needed surgery. Usually a hefty blow fractures a few ribs
after which sharp spicules of bone lacerate the surface
of spongy lungs. Blood, air or both then leak into the
chest cavity and the lung collapses proportionally. Most
penetrating wounds do the same. Usually all that is
needed is a plastic tube drain inserted between the ribs
and sucked on with a negative pressure machine. It's
a simple job of hoovering out the chest and allowing
the lung to fully expand again. Only if the blood clot
congeals into a solid mass so the drain cannot evacuate
it, do we operate. If we don't, the lung will never expand
and allow a full recovery. Unless the organs within
the chest are damaged, that just about sums up the
management of chest injuries except for the vital issue
of pain relief. I've had fractured ribs playing rugby. They
are absolute agony for a while.

Unsurprisingly, severe injuries to the heart and major
blood vessels hold a particular fascination for me, so
let me tell you about some cases where the innovative
technology I use daily in my career can save lives in

trauma patients. More often than not, the knife and gunshot wounds that survive to reach hospital are just holes that need closing. Evacuate the blood around the heart, a couple of carefully placed stitches and we're done. No heart-lung machine required. Most victims are young men who recover quickly and go on to more mischief.

Blunt injuries can be considerably more complex. As a piece of muscle full of blood under pressure the heart really doesn't enjoy a battering. The effects can directly replicate a heart attack but instead of myocardial infarction we call it myocardial contusion. And it causes an immediate drop in blood flow.

Picture the heart in the centre of the chest directly behind the breast bone and in front of the spine. In a high speed injury, particularly in an unrestrained driver, the heart can be compressed between them, suffering forces directly proportional to the speed of the vehicle and inversely related to the stopping distance. That's the scientific way of saying the poor organ is pulped between two solid walls of bone with the thin right ventricle at the front taking the brunt of the blow. Most patients in these circumstances show patchy areas of dead muscle and bleeding into the heart wall yet, in the setting of multiple trauma, cardiac injury is virtually always overlooked at first assessment. Ironic, then, that my first spectacularly life-threatening case was nothing to do with deceleration trauma. It was a bizarre one off.

The sixty-four-year-old carpenter was sharpening tools on a lathe when the spinning stone broke free from its bearings at speed. The heavy stone disc hit the man like a sledge hammer in the very centre of his

TO MEND A BROKEN HEART

chest leaving a circular bruise and knocking him from his feet in the process. When he arrived in the accident department he was semi-conscious in profound shock with distended neck veins which spelled out cardiac tamponade. I opened his left chest in the Emergency room, cut into the pericardium to drain the blood and right there was a rent in the apex of the high pressure left ventricle. As clots accumulated in the restricted space and the blood pressure fell precipitously, the bleeding had controlled itself. A couple of Teflon-buttressed stitches through the muscle edges and it was sorted. He survived because no one altered the precarious balance on the way to hospital, and he arrived quickly. Attempts at pre-hospital resuscitation would have killed him. His injury was very similar to a ruptured heart after a full thickness myocardial infarction, a condition that often results in sudden death.

Not long after that I was called to see a three-year-old girl who had been kicked in the chest by a horse on her parents' farm. Despite the unpleasantness of the incident, her injuries appeared to be restricted to bruising over the chest wall and, after a precautionary night in the children's ward, she was allowed home. Six days later she became listless and notably short of breath, seemingly without good reason. But when the GP listened to her chest he was immediately alarmed by a harsh heart murmur. The poor girl was brought back to hospital where an echo scan showed a thin layer of fluid around the heart but, more importantly, a discrete hole between the two pumping chambers which had not been present on the first admission. This is what we call a traumatic ventricular septal defect. The vicious blow had caused a localised heart attack just as occurs

THE TRAUMA CHRONICLES

in adults and the patch of dead muscle had given way to produce a hole in the heart.

It wasn't the right thing to operate immediately as we had done for the carpenter. A three-year-old heart is still quite small and newly dead muscle doesn't hold stitches well. So the cardiologists lessened her breathlessness with diuretics (water pills) water pills for six weeks then I opened her up to close the defect when the traumatised disintegrating muscle territory had been strengthened by scar tissue. Easily done by maintaining her circulation with the heart-lung machine and stopping the heart in a relaxed state with cold concentrated potassium solution. Then the hole was closed with a Dacron patch the size of a 10p piece. Straightforward and satisfying. Happily, she did just fine but keeps away from horses now.

These were both very unusual cases. In contrast, road traffic accidents are a frequent occurrence, yet severe injuries to the heart needing urgent surgery are also a rarity. Why? Because the victims often die before reaching hospital. A pulped heart doesn't last too long, but I seemed to attract them. One such patient was a thirty-five-year-old motorist who crashed headlong into the rear of a broken down lorry on the inside lane of a motorway near Oxford. Unrestrained, he suffered high velocity impact of the breast bone against the steering wheel, but neither breast bone nor ribs were broken. Fortuitously, as it transpired, he was admitted to hospital because of a leg fracture and minor head injury. Besides discomfort and bruising, no significant chest injuries were discovered at that time but five days later he complained of breathlessness with an unusually fast heart rate.

When the orthopaedic houseman used his stethoscope he could hear a loud precordial murmur which the

TO MEND A BROKEN HEART

cardiologists were asked to investigate. An echo scan then showed a severely leaking mitral valve in the left side of the heart, together with a dilated, poorly-contracting right ventricle immediately behind the breast bone. The sinister findings suggested severe blunt injury to the muscular septum between the two pumping chambers involving the small muscle that arises from there to support the mitral valve. It was a similar injury to the young girl kicked in the chest by the horse but with different manifestations.

The cardiologists tried to improve matters with water pills but without symptomatic improvement, so I was asked to explore the valve with a view to repairing it. But when I put him on the heart-lung machine, stopped the heart and inspected the valve it looked normal. It was the functional mechanism, the traumatised sub-valvar support pillar, that was impaired not the anatomy of the valve leaflets. Not wishing to remove a normal looking valve I made an effort to repair it by making the orifice smaller, hoping that the supporting muscle might recover with time. It didn't. There was little symptomatic improvement, the valve still leaked, and when the water tablets were reduced the patient's lungs filled with fluid again. I had no other option than to open him again a week later and replace the malfunctioning valve with a mechanical one for which he needed lifelong anticoagulant drugs. After that he recovered rapidly, had no further symptoms but was left wishing he had used that seat belt. And if I sound like a seat belt salesman I'm not. I just don't want to see young folk die when it can be avoided.

Just to reinforce the point, consider the case of a nineteen-year-old 'boy racer' in similar circumstances.

The lad was speeding along a two lane country road in the evening when he was forced to swerve abruptly to avoid a deer. The vehicle hit a solid oak tree at high speed and it was several minutes before he was found unconscious but breathing, while bleeding from head and facial wounds. There was no invasive pre-hospital care, thankfully. Once in hospital, the picture was dominated by the head injury and irrespective of bruising over the chest wall from steering wheel impact, the chest X-ray was thought to be normal. The following day, now conscious and disconnected from the breathing machine, he became agitated and complained of chest discomfort. This was attributed to bruising and it wasn't until the bright intensive care nurse brought attention to the rapid heart rate and border line blood pressure of 90/60 mm Hg that alarm bells started to ring. Though the electrocardiogram trace on the bedside monitor appeared innocuous, a formal six-lead electrocardiograph showed the classical pattern of a full blown heart attack. Five days after the accident, when his pain persisted, a heart catheter investigation was performed and opaque dye shot into the coronary arteries. The appearances were alarming. There was a 'blow out' like a balloon at the origin of the main vessel supplying his left ventricle. It was filled with blood clot with only sluggish flow beyond that point. What's more, the contraction of the heart muscle in the dependant territory was worryingly diminished. Diagnosis? The violent smack on the chest had damaged an important coronary artery and caused a major heart attack in a nineteen-year-old.

I was asked what I thought could be done about it. The obvious answer was a coronary bypass operation in case the vital vessel blocked off altogether. I planned to mobilise an artery from within the chest wall and join it to the damaged coronary beyond the blockage. This is a branch that arises from the main vessel to the left arm that we call the internal mammary artery because it supplies the breasts in women. You might be curious to know what happens to the breast if you do the same for a female. Does it turn black and fall off? Simple answer is no. Many arteries join together on the chest wall so others take over. A wonderful thing, the human body.

When I bisected his breast bone to dissect out the artery it was surrounded by bruising but still had a good flow. I didn't even put him on the bypass machine or stop his heart to do it. We were in the process of pioneering coronary bypass operations 'off pump' in those days and I'd organised the first big international meeting to teach the techniques right here in Oxford. It proved too intimidating for many of the attendants, particularly the American surgeons who constantly had the legal system on their backs. Yet others adopted the concept which conveyed substantial money-saving benefits. After all, heart-lung machines and those needed to run them are very expensive.

Did 'off pump' coronary bypass achieve the same results as the standard approach? Mostly, and it did for my injured patient. The renewed blood supply perked up the struggling heart muscle and he had no more pain. When I saw him months later in the outpatient clinic he was proud to announce that he had worn his seat belt on the way to the hospital. Most coronary bypass patients come along and tell me they have stopped smoking. Remarkable what a saw up the sternum can achieve.

THE TRAUMA CHRONICLES

Needless to say, the worst chest trauma I encountered came from motor cycle accidents. Their riders have little protection, tend to sustain multiple injuries, and many don't survive even after reaching hospital alive. Isolated cardiac injuries are rare in motorcyclists but do happen.

An eighteen-year-old woman wearing a helmet and leathers lost control in the rain and skidded into a concrete gate post. Though fully conscious with no apparent head injury or limb fractures, she became acutely short of breath, then pale, sweaty and cold. Seemingly in shock she was transferred by helicopter to the Oxford Trauma Unit without delay. There, during examination in the Emergency room, a loud heart murmur was heard. The chest X-ray performed soon after admission was abnormal and unusual. Both lungs were opaque with fluid and the heart shadow noticeably enlarged.

Despite the alarming picture there did not appear to be broken ribs or sternum, or free air or blood in the chest cavities. Suspecting a significant injury to the dilated heart, the cardiologists were called to perform a portable echo scan and my team were put on alert. It was mid-afternoon so I delayed sending for the next routine case of the day just in case. It was fortunate that we took that precaution. The young woman was deteriorating inexorably and had to be intubated and ventilated before any further investigations. When that happened, blood-stained froth spewed out of the tube in her windpipe.

The echocardiography was dramatic and unexpected. Indeed no one had seen anything like it before, nor heard of it happening. There was a hole in the root of her aorta, that main blood vessel supplying the whole body, just as it emerged from the heart above the valve. Normally such a rent would be immediately fatal, but in this case the vessel had burst through into the right atrium, the collecting chamber that receives blood from the body before the right ventricle pumps it through the lungs. Now the high pressure left side of the circulation was flooding the right and, as a result, the right atrium and ventricle were enormously dilated and tense. The traumatised right ventricle was barely contracting, just fluttering aimlessly. So the poor girl's diagnosis was a traumatic fistula between the left and right sides of the heart, now flooding the lungs and destined to prove fatal in a very short time. Had she not been brought into a cardiac surgical centre so quickly she would have stood no chance.

I watched the echocardiogram being performed with disbelief and summoned my fine anaesthetic colleague Kate to come and see the problem for herself. By then, there were indications that the patient had suffered a heart attack, too. Fundamentally we needed to get her onto the heart-lung machine as soon as possible to maintain the circulation and protect her watery lungs. So I wheeled her down the corridor from Emergency room to operating theatres myself. It took about 20 minutes to insert the appropriate transfusion and monitoring lines then the ubiquitous catheter into the bladder. As we expected there was little urine which, as we know, tells us that the kidneys, deprived of blood flow, weren't doing anything.

Once on the operating table, prepped and draped, it took little more than five minutes to make the incision, run the saw up the sternum, then zip open the pericardial sac to display my favourite organ. Or second favourite

THE TRAUMA CHRONICLES

as Woody Allen would have it. It happened that the pericardium had already split on impact causing a 15 cm rent down its right side with the distended atrium herniated through it. From a cardiac surgeon's perspective, on a scale of 0 to 10, this injury was a 9, with 10 proving fatal.

I went onto the bypass machine by putting a cannula directly into the aorta several centimetres above the damage, then two pipes directly into the main caval veins entering the right side of the heart. Had I made a hole directly into the tense, thin-walled right atrium it would probably have split spontaneously. Once the bypass machine was turned on it emptied out the right side of the heart, then a clamp between the perfusion cannula and the defect below gave us peace and tranquillity. For now she was safe, with plenty of time to achieve a repair, but I hadn't seen the damage yet.

The obvious finding was a tense purple collection of clotted blood beneath the thin membrane, or epicardium as we call it, around the root of the aorta. In essence this had placed a sticking plaster over the defect and prevented sudden death on site. This bruising extended along the pathway of the right coronary artery as it emerged adjacent to the fistula. From the dusky purple colour of the right ventricle, I surmised that the right coronary itself was completely occluded. That would account for the marked dilatation of the right ventricle and its vanishingly poor contraction. The muscle was dying. The Grim Reaper was perched on my shoulder at that point in time but my excitement was mounting.

As I've said before, operating on the unexpected in a trauma case is like opening a present at Christmas. Full

TO MEND A BROKEN HEART

of surprises, and I wasn't disappointed. When I opened the root of the aorta I found a small tear above the origin of that right coronary. But when I explored the right atrium separately to locate the corresponding entry hole I found the most curious and worrying of injuries. It was as if the very centre of the heart had split way down into the muscular septum between the pumping chambers. What's more, the tricuspid valve between the right atrium and ventricle was bisected by the tear and was leaking badly. All told this was a serious challenge. A bloody nightmare, in fact, but I was enjoying the challenge. Revelling in it, like being determined to win a computer game. Except I had never used a computer.

I considered the shredded right coronary artery as not repairable and I judged that tricuspid valve to be a write off too. Whatever I chose to do it was imperative not to destroy the invisible electrical conducting system in that split septum otherwise she would need a permanent pacemaker. So I replaced the torn tricuspid valve with a pig prosthesis using my Teflon-buttressed anchoring stitches to simultaneously close the rent in the muscle. Then I bypassed the occluded coronary artery with a segment of vein my registrar had dissected out from the girl's thigh. Having done that it was a simple matter to repair the fistula both from inside the aorta and within the right atrium. The whole process took around 65 minutes while the bypass machine provided blood flow to her body and brain. Very satisfying team work. Cardiologists, surgeons, anaesthetists, perfusionists and nursing staff all coming together to save a life. It's what we do.

Thankfully it all worked and the right ventricle with its new blood supply recovered in days. She was very

THE TRAUMA CHRONICLES

lucky to survive but, to re-emphasise, arriving quickly at the right hospital was the key.

As complex and taxing as it may seem, repairing hearts is what I did for a living. And as boring as it might seem, it was my hobby too, together with writing about it. Dramatic pictures from these cases are there to be seen in my textbooks. They made for compelling lectures too.

Sadly, it's not all happy endings at the sharp end. My very next trauma case was a thirty-eight-year-old motorcyclist who crashed at speed. He arrived unconscious with barely perceptible pulse and blood pressure and was tubed and ventilated immediately. The X-ray showed both lungs to be contused with free air in the left chest cavity, but of greater significance the cardiac shadow was distinctly abnormal with the apex of the heart elevated. By the time I reached the Emergency room he had received a couple of litres of fluid which failed to make any difference whatever to the blood pressure. Even vigorous external cardiac massage couldn't make a difference.

I knew precisely what the X-ray showed from bitter experience. It was another burst pericardial sac with the ventricles herniated and obstructed. Strangulated hearts can't fill and don't pump so he was unlikely to respond to resuscitation given the critically poor coronary blood flow since the accident. But as Winston said, 'Never, never, never give in,' so I opened his chest there and then on the trolley.

It was not a pretty sight, with the purple swollen ventricles protruding miserably from their fibrous bag. Starved of oxygen they were twitching agonally and about to die. But we still went through the motions.

226

I forced a finger through the defect and slit the sac wide open. With that the heart went still and gave up the ghost. Putting my right palm around the limp muscle I started to pump frantically and asked for a syringe of adrenaline. There was some bleeding from the chest wall for the first time so the cardiac massage was doing something.

I shot the adrenaline directly into the apex of the left ventricle so that it would hit the coronary arteries immediately. Sure enough the muscle stiffened and started to fibrillate lazily like a bag of worms. A few more vigorous squeezes and the tone improved so I asked for the defibrillating paddles. I told Rees, the anaesthetist, to administer sodium bicarbonate to neutralise acid in the blood stream then some calcium to perk up the heart muscle. Then I zapped it with 20 joules of direct electrical current in an attempt to restore a rhythm compatible with life. Nothing. The heart stopped dead again while his spinal muscles went into spasm causing him to rise abruptly from the trolley.

I decided to try one more shot of adrenaline to provoke the buggered heart but that also has disadvantages. It causes the arterial system to constrict, thereby increasing the resistance against which it has to pump should we get it started again. Again, the ventricles switched to fibrillation mode and I began to massage them, getting a feel for the tone and the right time to shock again. It's an experience thing. When you handle hearts every working day it becomes instinctive. So when it felt right I zapped the ventricles again. Ten joules first. That didn't do it. Up to 20 joules. *Zap*.

The ventricles stood still, flat lining, then a single spontaneous contraction. In a few seconds another one,

THE TRAUMA CHRONICLES

and then a short run of heart rhythm. Optimism for a few seconds then—shit! Fibrillation again, so another shot of 20 joules, and back to normal rhythm. At that point I asked for an intravenous shot of the local anaesthetic agent, lignocaine. This has a membrane-stabilising effect and helps to prevent ventricular dysrhythmia. And by now the fragile organ was starting to eject blood with blips on the pressure trace.

Now was the time to step back and watch patiently, hoping that it would keep going. The purple discoloration had disappeared but it was clear to me that the muscle had been damaged by the original blow. The right ventricle was barely contracting and we couldn't elevate the blood pressure above 70 mm Hg. The only sensible thing to do was to close the chest as quickly as possible, wheel him round to intensive care unit and insert what we call an 'intra-aortic balloon pump' to assist the circulation.

The device is just what it says on the box: a long sausage shaped balloon, rhythmically inflated then deflated by helium gas to reduce the amount of work the left ventricle has to do. Sadly, it doesn't pump much blood. We needed a different system for that known as 'extra corporeal membrane oxygenation' or ECMO, that I had pioneered for the UK, but the NHS wouldn't pay for it even in heart surgery centres and my 'freebies' had run out. Many Coronavirus patients needed ECMO during the pandemic but the whole of the UK could only manage a total of thirty circuits in five hospitals. Desperately disappointing as it was proven to save lives.

Death is cheap, and die he did, a couple of days later from heart failure. He never woke from his head injury. Miserably, I watched his wife and two daughters grieve by the bedside as he faded away. What can you say in those circumstances? 'We tried very hard, but despite our best efforts....'

I would like to believe that these heart trauma patients each received the best efforts of a major teaching hospital staffed by trauma enthusiasts. Willett's initiative to have senior surgeons in residence throughout the day and night had far reaching implications in that the emergency services were better organised. As in my own department, the nurses and ancillary staff took on advanced roles that created energy and enthusiasm for the job in hand. But at that stage, the rest of the NHS was still struggling to progress the proposal that patients with serious injuries should be managed by senior doctors, not disinterested waifs and strays who happened to be resident in the hospital.

By the turn of the century, the National Trauma Audit Research Network, whose job it was to monitor progress in the first NHS trauma centres, showed no significant change in the country overall. Though the likelihood of death following injury fell marginally between 1989 and 1994 there was no improvement after that. Still no more than 40% of seriously injured patients were treated by a consultant grade medic. Think about it. Why was our health care system vaunted as the 'envy of the world?'

RIGHT PLACE, RIGHT TIME

The boundaries between life and death are
shadowy and vague. Who shall say where the one
ends and where the other begins?

Edgar Allan Poe

The handover from the ambulance crew was worrying.

We have a young woman with gunshot wounds
to the chest and abdomen. When we picked her
up she was screaming 'my baby, my baby' and
she does look as if she's heavily pregnant. We
can't get a blood pressure on the cuff but there's a
faint carotid pulse in her neck. Over the last few
minutes she's not responding anymore.

Knife and gunshot wounds were a daily occurrence in that
hospital. It was a concise and revealing report but I didn't
understand a word of it. The dialogue was in Portuguese.
On the final morning of a visiting Professorship in Brazil
I was being shown around the huge city hospital by a
vivacious surgical resident called Leonor. I guessed that
she had been carefully selected to entertain the British
heart surgeon following his breakfast time talk. There
was little point in me attending the remainder of the
morning's presentations when I didn't speak the language.
Same old story. Everyone was expected to listen to me
lecturing in English after which I would take off.

THE TRAUMA CHRONICLES

As the thoracic surgeon on call, Leonor had been fast bleeped to the trauma room in advance of an arrival, and rather than return to the conference I went along with her in curiosity. In the midst of the handover the resuscitation efforts were beginning, so all I could see was frenetic activity within a curtained cubicle full of nurses and medical staff. Blood-stained underwear was cast off onto the floor. Doctors were barking orders, with nurses trying to fulfil them, so I coaxed my Latino consort to edge her way in. When someone calls for a chest surgeon urgently there is usually good reason or it. 'Come with me then,' she bleated nervously.

The woman was white as a sheet. Wide bore cannulas were being shoved skilfully into invisible collapsed veins in her arms and neck. Then, having lost consciousness already, the tracheal tube was deftly manoeuvred deep into the windpipe without sedation. That made her cough and, as she did, jets of purple blood spurted from bullet wounds in the chest. When oxygen was rhythmically hand blown in to her lungs, those incongruous fountains morphed into steady streams flowing around the contours of her swollen breasts.

Naked as she was now, the missile entry wounds were readily apparent. There were three of them in the chest, two to the right of the breast bone, one to the left, each above the nipple line. Then two more in the upper abdomen directly over the liver and dome of the pregnant uterus. That was particularly worrying. I couldn't help thinking it was intended for the baby's head.

Bags of uncrossed group O negative blood were kept in the Emergency room fridge for just this purpose. Two of them were squeezed in rapidly after which the carotid pulse could be felt in the neck. That suggested

RIGHT PLACE, RIGHT TIME

the blood pressure to be in the region of 60 mm Hg, half normal. Enough to keep her alive but not so good for the placenta and unborn baby. With a semblance of consciousness beginning to return, she became agitated, coughing up fresh blood through the tracheal tube.

From my own bitter experience and a clear three dimensional picture of the anatomy, I really didn't need X-rays or scans to illustrate what injuries had been inflicted. The fact that she had survived to this point gave me grounds for optimism. She may have lost a considerable amount of blood but it was not from the heart or a major blood vessel, otherwise she would have died rapidly at the scene. As we've said, some victims of penetrating heart wounds survive with cardiac tamponade and low blood pressure but her neck veins were not distended, nor did the entry wounds indicate that. From their location, and given the distortion of her anatomy through advanced pregnancy, I suspected the bleeding to come from the liver, both lungs and possibly a shattered placenta.

There was heated debate amongst the Emergency room doctors as to whether the woman should be rushed to the CT scanner. Again, I had no notion of what was being said in real time but Leonor kept translating the discussions for me. She had already informed them that I was a visiting heart surgeon and invited guest from the UK. What's more, given the imminent risk to life for mother and child, she insisted that they should listen to what I had to say. There was no other surgeon present and as a humble resident she felt uncomfortably out of her depth.

In Oxford I had built a practice of repairing the hearts of pregnant women on the heart-lung machine while preserving their babies. That was a tall order as many died and spontaneously aborted afterwards. I had published a seminal article on the subject in the American surgical literature and one aspect that I well understood was that heavily pregnant women were difficult to resuscitate. That is because of the obstructive compression of the major veins in the abdomen by the gravid uterus which can reduce circulating blood flow by as much as a third. So, to begin with, the woman in front of us would fare better tipped towards her left side, a manoeuvre which also relieves compression of the base of the larger right lung. Small point but that simple change immediately made a positive difference to her blood pressure.

I also knew that the unborn infant and placental circulation are very sensitive to the blood vessel constricting drug adrenaline used routinely during resuscitation. Moreover blood oxygen levels must be kept as high as possible to protect the baby's brain. For that reason, I urged Leonor to get on and insert drains into each side of the chest to evacuate the blood and allow the compressed lungs to re-expand.

Emboldened by Leonor's introductory comments, I asked one of the Emergency room doctors to lend me her stethoscope. As anticipated I could barely hear breath sounds because of the collapsed lungs but that wasn't what I was listening for. I wanted to hear the infant's heartbeat. First to reassure us that it was still alive, but second so we might predict what damage to expect. If the head was sitting high in the uterus the bullets may have caused brain damage. But hopefully the head was down in the pelvis already, in which case the heartbeat should be lower down and the skull protected by the pelvic bones.

I could hear mother's heart sounds easily enough which essentially ruled out cardiac tamponade. Then happily I picked up faint, very rapid heart sounds just above her pubic bone. So a bullet traversing the dome of the uterus would have missed baby's head and chest. Clearly the infant was still alive. What's more, pressure from the stethoscope prompted a strong uterine contraction.

All this was pointing to one thing in my mind. Something that did not seem readily apparent to the assembled audience. The surest route to salvage both lives was to extricate that baby fast. It was only fair to verbalise those thoughts then shift into executive mode with Leonor's help. Everyone else seemed uncertain about what to do next—they were relatively inexperienced so who could blame them.

Although the transfusion had given the woman a measurable blood pressure it was not at a level to provide safety for the baby. The woman was still in shock with low blood oxygen levels and too much acid in the blood. That combination depresses cardiac function in both mother and child so I urged Leonor to insert those chest drains as soon as possible. She was clearly nervous so when I offered to do it myself, there came a tacit nod of acceptance from all involved—the medics seemed only too keen to relinquish responsibility for an alarmingly high risk situation.

I briefly wondered whether the barely conscious victim's level of awareness warranted the use of local anaesthetic. I didn't think so. So I took the scalpel and, as she lay on her left side, I shoved it through the right chest wall at the base of the armpit. That woke her up a bit, and I guess it was a bit much being stabbed and shot on the same morning. So I quickly followed

THE TRAUMA CHRONICLES

through with the drain itself on its sharp metal trocar. On withdrawing the introducer to connect the tubing, blue blood gushed out through the drain and onto the floor. Around half a litre of it before I succeeded in attaching everything where it belonged. The phrase 'better out than in' came to mind but would have been wasted in translation.

Having succeeded with the right chest I decided to move on to the left. The monitor showed that her blood pressure had risen to 80/60 mm Hg given the additional transfusion and change in position. Not surprisingly, my machinations had woken her up too, therefore it was no longer reasonable to stab her a second time without pain relief. But as we rolled her over to present the left chest uppermost she suddenly flat lined. The blood pressure disappeared altogether. Given the metabolic mayhem and a burst of her own adrenaline on waking, the heart muscle had fibrillated. Now there was just disordered electrical activity with the heart muscle squirming aimlessly instead of pumping. In other words, sudden death. The phrase 'shit and derision' drifted through my frontal lobes and I needed every ounce of psychopathy I could muster.

Once supine again, one of the interns launched into vigorous cardiac compressions as if his own life depended upon it. Crunch, crunch, crunch, forcefully dislocating rib cartilage from bone. Further disrupting the placenta. More trauma was the last thing the poor woman needed. The phrase 'shot, stabbed, now beaten to death,' morbidly came to mind. The pulverised heart just needed to be shocked back into normal rhythm and there was still time enough for that. Worse still, a second doctor was hovering with a syringe full of adrenaline.

Sure it would give a powerful boost to the mother's heart but it was potentially lethal for the placental circulation and the oxygen starved child imprisoned inside.

Was anyone confident enough to defibrillate a heavily pregnant woman with her full term baby? It was 'should we or shouldn't we?' 'What if the shock stopped the baby's heart?' The committee couldn't make up its mind, but a full blown debate was not what the patient needed. Both their lives were drifting away through indecision and the increasing likelihood of a broken rib being pushed into the middle of the mother's right ventricle. As such, I felt compelled to intervene so discretion checked out as impulse kicked in.

With apologies to the poor child I took the defibrillating paddles and gave the mother a high voltage shock across the chest. Zap. Her spinal muscles went into spasm arching her back and lifting her from the trolley. I'm sure the uterus contracted too but the move had the desired effect. Her heart began to beat in a coordinated fashion and a blood pressure trace returned to the monitor screen.

With Leonor translating I made it clear to the medical staff that if she fibrillated again the baby must be delivered rapidly for both of their sakes. As anticipated, it was impossible to resuscitate the woman then operate on her wounds with that uterus obstructing the circulation. Leonor requested that they bring a tray of surgical instruments to the cubicle with gowns and gloves for us both. That baby needed to be taken out within four minutes of a further cardiac arrest, so last chance. Would anyone else care to take over? There was deafening silence as my words were translated into Portuguese.

A scalpel and vascular clamps was all I really needed, but if they had a bone saw for the breast bone that would be great. Needless to say they didn't, but unbridled impulsivity had taken over leaving little regard for place or circumstances. Daunting as it all may seem, to cut is to fix, and that came to me instinctively. Not slowly and deliberately, but fast and on autopilot in this case. Was this ruthless psychopathy coming to the fore in an unfamiliar environment, or just a caring surgeon doing his job? Difficult to tell.

I was not about to perform a standard caesarean section though a low transverse incision. My intention was to open her belly from top to bottom giving me simultaneous access to both baby and gunshot wounds. Why the four minute limit? The brain dies rapidly without blood flow and it would be impossible to extricate the infant and perform external cardiac massage at the same time. If needed, it would be 'no pissing about' surgery. More 'slash and grab.'

While all eyes followed the ECG and blood pressure trace on the monitor screen my gaze was fixed upon the abdomen full of baby and blood. I felt another powerful uterine contraction and noticed a pool of fresh blood between her thighs. While uterine muscle is highly elastic the placenta isn't. The crucial interface between the two is easily broken down. Either the bullet or forceful cardiac compressions must have triggered separation of the placenta with vaginal bleeding. A bloody disaster – literally.

At that point, the alarm on the monitor announced that her young heart had fibrillated again, the second cardiac arrest within ten minutes. That was the starting pistol. I had just a couple of minutes to cut the baby out of its hostile confinement before attempting to resuscitate mother in more favourable circumstances. This was pure objectivity. No ifs nor buts. The others were told to back off. No cardiac compressions, no defibrillation, no nothing until the child was out. I figured that four to five minutes without circulation was an acceptable pay off for the mother as long as her resuscitation efforts were well managed afterwards.

With hands visibly trembling, Leonor sprayed iodine solution over the protuberant belly from nipples to pubis. My scalpel followed, cutting deep and swerving sympathetically around an everted umbilicus. The pressure applied instinctively to the blade drove it down through skin and fat onto the fibrous membrane between the stretched rectus muscles of the abdominal wall. Cut carefully through that and there was a glimpse of the uterus. Like a rugby ball floating in a red pool. But with cardiac arrest there was no active bleeding, just spilled blood slopping around the abdominal cavity. I ignored it, choosing to extend the incision along the whole length of the belly. One minute gone.

Before me now was the dome of the muscular cocoon with its precious load; then the bullet hole bearing witness to a malevolent attempt to murder the unborn child. Was there a camera in the department to illustrate that fact? Sadly not but I could see and feel movement inside. Perhaps a response to the searing pain that heralded the child's miserable introduction to the world. And at that point I would have cheerfully slit the perpetrator's throat with my blade. So perhaps Dutton was right.

My career had witnessed many desperate battles with Grim Reaper. A few involved mother and child but never before when someone had deliberately tried to murder the innocent. This was new to me. My adrenaline was pumping, fingers flashing purposefully without conscious thought. They knew what to do. How deep to cut, how hard to retract, how cautiously to drag on the wounded child. I inserted the index finger of my left hand through the bullet hole and located it behind the placenta. That was good. The dense tissue had absorbed the velocity of the missile. What's more I could now zip open the uterine muscle by cutting down onto my own finger. Two minutes gone.

All too quickly a squirming loop of umbilical cord slithered out like a snake and happily I could feel a bounding pulse in it. The infant's blood pressure was clearly better than mother's and the head was indeed nestled down in the pelvis. Eager to meet it, I unzipped the womb like a sports bag. I could then pass my hand behind the baby's shoulders to lift it out. Slippery, profoundly blue and bloodstained, I didn't notice whether it was a boy or girl. A cruel and hideous wound to the right leg had drawn my attention. Three minutes gone.

An obstetrician was waiting behind me as Lenora clamped the cord and cut through it. Paranoid about dropping the precious bundle I turned carefully and placed it into a towel. Phase one of the struggle was complete. We were now four minutes into the mother's cardiac arrest so my efforts diverted quickly to provide a run of cardiac compressions. 'How much blood have you given her?' I quizzed the anaesthetist, who spoke English. 'Six units so far' he replied. 'I'm sure she needs more,' I insisted. 'And give her some bicarbonate and calcium. I'll try to defibrillate her, but if I have trouble I'm going to open her chest.'

I gave another run of compressions, attempting to push some oxygenated blood into her coronary arteries, then carefully positioning the defibrillating paddles over breast bone and left chest, I pushed the button. *Zap*, followed by brief flat lining then fibrillation again. After another run of forceful cardiac massage, I tried again. Same result. So I stood back for a moment's contemplation as Leonor took over the pumping. She was good at it. I could hear the ends of the fractured ribs grating against each other and that helped to focus my mind. The special forces have a saying—*if you're going through hell, keep going.*

'I need to open her chest now' I told the nurses, loud enough to regain the anaesthetists attention. He just stared at me, but wasn't going to object. I would have liked to run a saw straight up the breast bone as for all my heart operations, but as usual they didn't have one in the department. Amongst the instruments available was an old fashioned chest opening set so I opted for what we call a 'clam shell' incision. For a better chance of restarting this heart I literally needed it in my hands. Open cardiac massage is much more effective. It allows me to inject drugs directly into the left ventricle. Then palpating the muscle tone tells me when to shock it. All instinctive. I had just delivered a baby, but heart surgery was my day job.

As I set about carving a transverse incision beneath the swollen breasts I heard the baby cry for the first time. That sent out the most powerful of messages. Motivating in the extreme. And from the animated chatter behind me I gleaned it was a girl. I simply wasn't going to see her without a mother on the day she was born.

'Happy birthday, little mouse,' I murmured quietly.

By now I was sweating like a pig. Cutting between the ribs on each side of the breast bone, I slipped a finger through into both chest cavities. As expected, frothy blood and air came pissing out as I made a tunnel between the two, then chopped through the bone with an orthopaedic surgeon's chisel. Cranking wide that slit with a metal retractor created the 'clam shell' entering both chest cavities and exposing the pericardial sac. As predicted, the heart was intact. The missiles missed it. As far as I could see they had traversed the chest wall and spongy lung tissue but no major blood vessels. Lucky lady.

Opening the pericardium from top to bottom, I took the ventricles in my hand and used my fist as the pump until I could get them started again. When I squeeze the muscle in my palm I know instinctively whether the muscle tone is ready to shock or if the heart contains enough blood. It was still empty. She needed more transfusion and now, with the baby out, it was time to shoot in the adrenaline. I really didn't want to pulverise the poor organ for longer than necessary. A short lapse in concentration and a thumb or finger could find itself inside the chambers. That event usually terminates the resuscitation efforts.

The syringe of hope was waiting. Lifting the squirming muscle towards me through the incision, I slid the needle into the apex of the left ventricle and shot in the stimulant. A couple of manual squeezes and adrenaline reached the coronary arteries. The response to the hormone was instantaneous. Like pouring petrol on flames. The ventricles stiffened and squirmed angrily like a sack of hungry rats. Now was the time to shoot. *Zap*.

Just 20 joules halted the fibrillation allowing the heart to beat again in coordinated fashion. I dropped it like a hot potato as vigorous pressure waves appeared on the screen. Better still, it looked good to me. On the runway and preparing to take off again. Even the bright red bleeding from the wound edges was a welcome site.

So far I had seen nothing to convince me that the wounds would prove fatal. There was low velocity bullet damage to the fragile liver and both lungs but no profuse bleeding that was difficult to control. Neither could I detect the odour of perforated bowel that might lead to infection. It was biochemistry, not bullets, that was the problem by now, nor was an Emergency room bay the right place to put everything back together again. That required a sterile operating environment, bright theatre lights and the appropriate surgical instruments.

My Heath Robinson rescue efforts in suit trousers and surgical gown had kept them both alive, but now they deserved better. With perspiration soaking my shirt, my parting gift was some well-placed stitches through the bullet holes in the lungs which reduced the bleeding to a trickle. Then some dry packs over the holes in the liver. Liver doesn't stitch well. Blood clotting does the job better.

Inevitably, a crowd had assembled outside the resuscitation bay, many of them wearing operating theatre scrubs. Some were caring for the newborn girl and her wounds. Others belonged to the on call surgical team who had been at my lecture and summoned from the conference to help. I sensed it was the right time to let them take over. To get the mother into an operating

THE TRAUMA CHRONICLES

theatre where the obstetricians could remove the remains of the placenta and put the uterus back together. Leonor could do her bit by closing the huge incisions and the frazzled anaesthetist could hand over to a substitute then recover from his nervous breakdown.

The young are resilient. I felt both mother and baby would make it now. So stepping backwards I asked my beautiful assistant 'would you take over now Leonor? It's time for me to go. I have a plane to catch. If I leave you my mobile number it would be kind if you would call to let me know how things turn out.' She gave me an anxious glare, wide eyed above the mask. As if to say 'you have to be joking!' But I wasn't. I should have set off for the airport already. I had been in South America for two weeks and was desperate to get home. But in the midst of the excitement, I had lost track of time.

The 18.50 British Airways 747 was waiting on the tarmac, an upstairs seat in Business Class booked in my name. But now there was a snag. Out in the real world, torrential rain had brought the outskirts of the sprawling city to a standstill. Worse still, the tropical deluge had flooded the airport highway underpass. Now nothing could pass. Had I set off in good time I would simply have been caught in miles of traffic already backed up to the centre of town. Now it was check in time and I was still in the hospital.

One of Leonor's canny resident colleagues offered to help out. His family lived close to the airport so he knew uncharted backroads through the favelas and would do his utmost to get me there. It was time to depart at top speed. My parting words? 'Thanks for your help, Leonor. Take good care of them both. I'm sure you're going to make a great cardiac surgeon.' I caught a glimpse of the baby as I walked away. Her left leg below the knee was shattered by the bullet. The foot was purple so I feared its blood supply to be compromised but that was not my business now. At least she was alive and wailing loudly.

The rainy dash to the airport was not straightforward. The streets were awash and there was poor visibility through the windscreen. Several attempted routes were aborted but finally he got me there half an hour after take-off time. I knew that I had missed the flight and set about considering the increasingly dismal options. Should I stay the night at the airport or venture back to my hotel in the city?

First I needed to rebook the flight for the following evening but I was surprised to find the check in desk was still open. I thought that unusual had the flight already departed. It turned out that it hadn't. The flight crew were also stuck in the flood and hadn't arrived yet. The latest update was that they were still half an hour away. Then there would be another half an hour's preparation time before boarding and take-off. 'You're one of the lucky ones, Sir,' the receptionist said. 'Most of the passengers are well and truly stuck and won't make it. You'll virtually have the plane to yourself. Please enjoy the lounge next to the gate and we'll call you in good time.'

The airport lounge was virtually empty as I sat with a bottle of red wine and a large bowl of nuts staring through a rainy window. Seeing nothing. Homicide in pregnant women was not uncommon in South America but it certainly was in Oxford. At home, my heart operations on heavily gravid women were all carefully planned and orchestrated. The operation that day was opportunistic and impulsive. Done purely on instinct

THE TRAUMA CHRONICLES

in desperation. I quietly revisited it all in my mind. Convention dictates 'Save the mother at the expense of the unborn infant.' But it was virtually impossible to resuscitate a woman by cardiac compressions with a heavy uterus compressing the abdominal veins. Add to that the wounded baby and a bleeding placenta. So bugger convention. Get on and save both.

As I poured another large glass of sedative at the bar my mobile rang. I had given Leonor my number and hoped it was her. Not from anything but a professional standpoint, I might add—as attractive as she was, my philandering days had long past by then.

'Hi Prof, I gather that you made it to the airport but missed the plane. Do you want to come back into town and go out with us residents for dinner? We'd love to treat you.'

'Leonor, I was late but the plane is still here' I replied. The crew were later than I was. 'I would have loved to have dinner with you,' secretly wishing it was just the two of us, 'but I'm about to board. Dare I ask how the patients are?'

'Oh they're both doing fine. By the time we got to theatre the bleeding from the lungs had stopped. There was still oozing from the liver so we left packs in the abdomen. The obstetricians sewed up the uterus and they seem happy with the baby. A vascular surgeon is looking at the leg right now. We can't thank you enough, Prof. Without you there we would have lost them both. Now it looks as if both will make it.'

I was silent and a tad emotional, given that last sentence. I decided to be a surgeon in the backstreets of Scunthorpe because I wanted to make a difference. That day I had made a difference in the drenched favelas of Sau Paulo, a very long way from home. So I asked lovely Leonor to keep me posted. Then I added the obvious 'I couldn't have done it without your help so go off with your friends and celebrate. Then think about coming over to train with me.'

Throughout my career, happiness was a night flight home on the upper deck of a 747. My seat was the only one occupied. It was like a private club up there. Two flight attendants, one passenger and a fully stocked drinks trolley. It was before 9/11 and the doors of the flight deck were open. I watched the pilots going through their check list and wondered why surgeons didn't live by the same rules. Some years later, the World Health Organisation did indeed introduce surgical check lists for operating theatres.

As usual, I had neglected to switch off my mobile phone as we pushed back from the gangway. There was a ping, this time heralding a text message. *Mother has woken up already. Brain seems to be fine. Baby stable but still in theatre. Never forget today.* Then three final words that made me smile. *Or you, Prof!*

Taking off in the deluge was not a problem and, once above the clouds, it was plain sailing. The first question from the stewardess was always the same.

'How was your trip, Sir?'

Did I want to play the heart surgeon card that night. Not at all. So I just said 'very wet, I'm afraid. I'm pleased to be going home.' Then more red wine, this time of better quality.

Without doubt, my involvement in that case as an onlooker was both impulsive and reckless. It could have easily gone the other way and resulted in two tragic deaths. But without intervention both would be in a mortuary fridge now, lying together in the cold and dark. As that iconic monster of an aeroplane rumbled

THE TRAUMA CHRONICLES

through the sky, I looked back on the fact that my whole career had been 'off piste.' That's why I had pissed off so many people. Many of the initiatives that defined Oxford cardiac surgery and changed the specialty for the better were much criticised by the usual suspects. First came the 'cardiac surgery without intensive care' strategy. A fast track recovery programme which we needed because there were never enough critical care beds. Then we introduced surgical nurse practitioners to harvest leg veins for coronary bypass surgery because the transient trainee surgeons didn't always make a good job of it. That caused cataclysmic eruptions in both the Royal College of Nursing and Royal College of Surgeons. Next we started a new paediatric cardiac surgery programme that ruffled feathers. Then we pioneered new mechanical circulatory support devices both in the laboratory and clinic. That resulted in Oxford becoming the first cardiac unit the in world to implant a permanent high speed rotary blood pump as an alternative to a heart transplant. It transpired that the pumps worked well providing equivalent survival without the complications of immunosuppressive drugs at a time when seat belts greatly reduced the numbers of organ donors. And as I always said, no treatment that relies exclusively on someone else to die first can ever fulfil the requirement. Blood pumps can.

Irrespective of the fact that all of these schemes paid off handsomely with great benefit to patients worldwide, they were a constant risk to my own reputation in Britain. Having said that, I thrived on conflict and consider that our innovation in cardiothoracic surgery made an important contribution to one of Britain's first major trauma centres.

Trauma of a Different Kind

It looks as if the NHS will gradually fade away,
and we shall go back to a great deal of private
medicine

Ruth Rendell

Trauma comes in different guises and, fittingly for the last stage of my career, I was about to interface closely with one of the most traumatic events the world had yet to experience. It had been a full forty years since my adventures at Harefield when I arrived in Wuhan, on 19 December 2019. After a long overnight flight I was in the habit of taking a walk to blow away the cobwebs. I could never succumb to jet lag, there wasn't the time. Just yards in front of the hotel was a walkway on the bank of the Yangtze River with its spectacular bridge, much like the Golden Gate in San Francisco. For the most part I loved being in China. I'd always had spooky memories of my first adventure there in 1978 immediately after Mao's Cultural Revolution. I'd been operating as a locum general surgeon in Hong Kong and gained access to a large hospital in Guangzhou courtesy of Colonel Bob Stewart, the head of MI6. I never expected to see heart surgery on patients still awake and without a ventilator. The hospital simply didn't have any ventilators. How did I get involved with MI6? That's another story.

THE TRAUMA CHRONICLES

Wuhan is a bustling metropolis of eleven million people packed into an astonishing density of high rise residential tower blocks. It had been freezing in Oxford so the balmy subtropical air was appealing, yet there was little traditional Chinese culture on view. At least until I reached the gates of the notorious Huanan Seafood Market. As an animal lover I found the place deeply distasteful. Beyond the seafood there were dogs, cats, snakes and bats in abundance, either cramped in small cages or dead then brutally butchered. Then there were pangolins, unusual creatures that played a crucial role in what came next.

The novel new virus had not been characterised as yet. Nor was there wide knowledge of it as I meandered through the colourful stalls that afternoon. A hypothesis under consideration was that it had spread from bats to pangolins then on to humans in that very market. Others would soon suggest that sinister experiments at the Wuhan Institute of Virology was a better bet. That wasn't far away either. Scientists there were researching the relationships between a variety of coronaviruses and bats in the caves of rural China. But to what end? Perhaps the world was about to find out.

It was the huge annual meeting of the Chinese Association of Cardiothoracic Surgery and a particular honour to present the opening address to three thousand attendees. That said, I was booked on a flight back to Heathrow the same afternoon in time for Christmas with the family. So when a group of surgeons, hospital administrators and intensive care doctors approached me after the talk it was unexpected. At first they stood their silently waiting for me to sign copies of the Chinese edition of *Fragile*

TRAUMA OF A DIFFERENT KIND

Lives. They were all wearing masks but I was familiar with that in China and Japan.

The tone was serious. Would I discuss a worrying development with them? Amongst other mechanical circulatory support systems, I had talked about extracorporeal membrane oxygenation (ECMO), and the fact that I had used it successfully in Oxford during the British swine flu outbreak. In particular it had saved one particular child with uncorrected congenital heart disease who was otherwise certain to die. My inquisitors were curious to understand whether it could be deployed safely for other types of severe viral pneumonia, and of course the rest is history. They had encountered around fifty cases in the city at the time but in reality there were several hundred and the patients were dying from respiratory failure. Positive pressure ventilation was causing further damage to the fragile inflamed lung tissue.

I suggested that I might review a patient before deciding, but with that they went quiet.

'The problem is being kept under wraps,' one surgeon replied in perfect English. 'But we wanted to ask your advice when we saw you on the programme.'

Having satisfied them, I was handed a plate with a picture of their hospital on it and a box of Chinese tea. After shaking hands vigorously I departed to find some traditional dolls for my granddaughters, then my flight home beckoned. A short, and as it turned out, an eventful trip.

It was mid-January when I received a polite follow up call from the conference organisers who were curious to know whether I had been ill? I hadn't but my wife and son certainly had two weeks after I arrived home.

By then, Covid-19 had its name and would become familiar to virtually every person in the world. China had ordered a draconian lockdown of Hubei Province enforced by police and the military. I received pictures of the vast conference hall, which was now home to several hundred makeshift hospital beds. Moreover, Wuhan built a huge new Covid isolation hospital in just two weeks and were soon running fifty ECMO systems continuously for their sickest patients. When their locally manufactured ECMO circuits were exhausted, they began importing systems from Germany.

I kept in contact with my Chinese colleagues in the coming weeks as the shocking facts of the epidemic emerged. Many doctors and nurses were infected by their patients and died. Yet, in the meantime, the thrice weekly flights from Wuhan to Heathrow kept coming, long after Hong Kong had closed its borders. Welcome to Terminal 4. Eventually it was the Chinese Government who suspended all air and rail departures from Wuhan on 23 January. Ours sat back watching to see what would happen.

A pattern of illness emerged whereby 85% of patients suffered mild to moderate symptoms of fever, cough and fatigue which seemingly resolved over a couple of weeks. However, the remainder progressed to suffer severe breathlessness, initially attributable to viral pneumonia but occurring eight to ten days after the initial onset. Standard treatments with oxygen therapy or mechanical ventilation failed to save the majority of these patients, raising questions about the true nature of the lung pathology. This late stage disease just didn't behave like straightforward viral pneumonia as other organs failed rapidly too. And the virus was spreading like wild fire.

Given the ominous contagion and prohibitive mortality of Covid, the Chinese steered away from performing autopsies. It happened that the characteristic pathology was described incidentally in an asymptomatic Covid patient who had a lung removed for cancer. Though the patient wasn't sick there were still diffuse patches of pulmonary infection consisting of oedematous tissue crammed with white blood cells. Inflammatory markers called cytokines were substantially raised in the patient's blood and the smallest airways were blocked by sticky plugs of proteinaceous material. They were being asphyxiated and oxygen introduced by the breathing machine simply didn't enter the blood stream.

Three factors taken in combination seemed to portend fatal Covid. The first was a rise of liver enzymes in the blood indicating multi-organ involvement. The second was an elevated haemoglobin level related to low blood oxygen levels over the previous weeks, and the third was generalised muscle pains known as myalgia.

The elderly male population were most susceptible to severe disease and those with pre-existing heart problems, high blood pressure and diabetes fared worse. That was because the virus entered the cells through latching on to 'so called' ACE receptors and, sure enough, the majority who died showed signs of inflammation in their heart muscle too. Many complained of palpitations, chest pain and dizziness unrelated to the respiratory illness. Others experienced damage to the lining of their blood vessels causing thrombosis, heart attacks or stroke.

The concept emerged in Wuhan that both the heart and lungs were under attack following massive cytokine release and what is known as a T cell immune response aimed at destroying the tissues containing the virus. In other words the virus wasn't killing the patient, their own immune system was. The time course of deterioration after initial mild symptoms seemed to support that case, with most of the deaths occurring through catastrophic multi-organ failure.

More and more of what I learned in those first weeks triggered alarm bells. Curiously, the life-threatening clinical picture vividly reminded me of the Post Perfusion Syndrome in the early days of the heart-lung machine. Foreign materials in the cardiopulmonary bypass circuit triggered complement activation then cytokine release in the blood that was followed by a lethal whole body inflammatory response in the patient. White blood cells clogged the small blood vessels in the lungs, kidneys and liver causing life-threatening functional impairment. There were so many similarities.

My long nights making those discoveries in the laboratory in Alabama came drifting back to me. Many infants and frail or elderly patients died from lung and kidney failure after we repaired their hearts simply because of blood foreign surface interaction and the cytokine storm that generated. What's more, prolonged periods on a positive pressure ventilator sealed their fate. Should that be the case for Covid, steroids might help to damp down the inflammation. That dawned upon me on Valentine's Day 2020, and I considered trying to share the suggestion.

Needless to say, my interest in the cardiovascular consequences of Covid extended beyond curiosity. The virus caused heart failure and I was developing a unique artificial heart that did not need an electric power cable exiting through the skin. Now it seemed the pandemic would decimate organ transplantation on a worldwide

TRAUMA OF A DIFFERENT KIND

basis. A realistic alternative would be needed, which I hoped would prove preferable to the complications of immunosuppression in the long term. I had one.

After operating on their heart, all of my patients left the operating theatre on a ventilator yet, throughout my whole career, I endeavoured to discontinue respiratory support as quickly as possible. Why? Because positive pressure ventilation is not a benign process and the deleterious effects are substantially worsened when the cellular lining of the lungs is under attack. In stiff oedematous lungs, both high levels of inflation pressure and high oxygen concentrations damage the fragile tissues. In turn, muscle-paralysing agents and strong sedative drugs given for long periods have serious effects on recovery. When it is time to attempt spontaneous breathing again, ventilated patients are debilitated by muscle weakness because recumbency alone causes a 10% loss of body muscle mass in 10 days. These issues resulted in an early intensive care mortality rate exceeding 80% in China, Italy and North America.

First to recognise the problem, the Chinese went to substantial lengths to avoid mechanical ventilation as their patients deteriorated. First they employed vapourised enzyme preparations to dissolve the mucus plugs clogging the airways. Then they used a mixture of hydrogen gas with oxygen to reduce the viscosity of the inhaled gases and diminish the effort of breathing. As well as reducing airways resistance, hydrogen had an anti-inflammatory effect which succeeded in keeping patients out of an intensive care bed.

I tried to convey my insights from China to colleagues in the NHS in a genuine effort to be helpful. Given the similarities between catastrophic Covid and the post perfusion syndrome, I suggested that steroids or a membrane stabiliser such as zinc, or even arsenic, might protect the failing organs. Unfortunately, the suggestion of giving an infected patient something to suppress the immune response was derided and I was ignored. The ramblings of a retired surgeon were deemed unhelpful and, while the Chinese were being blamed for the outbreak, their 'Oriental witchcraft' was considered of no interest.

Informing the Oxford intensive care doctors that positive pressure ventilation was going to make Covid lungs worse didn't help either. The hospital had adopted the government's tightly regulated research agenda which couldn't be challenged. When I told them about hydroxy gas machines, I was politely told to 'butt out.'

Worse was yet to come. Westminster's knee jerk response to a tsunami of infected patients was to create thousands of new critical care beds by shutting down other services. These were equipped with rapidly manufactured basic ventilators placed in the hands of volunteer medical staff, many of whom were surgeons made redundant by the discontinuation of their practice. The 'ventilators and volunteers' initiative was an appropriate description. Ill-informed at best, lethal in practice.

Instead of ordering more regulatory approved breathing machines, the Health Secretary elected to spend £50 million with diverse engineering companies to develop the most basic models that could be rolled out quickly. These were delivered into the hands of untrained staff given just a couple of days instruction. According to the regulator, at least twelve ventilators produced with urgency were simply too risky to use.

TRAUMA OF A DIFFERENT KIND

Having negotiated personally with the Prime Minister, Sir James Dyson wasted £20 million in his efforts. Incidentally, when we sought his help to improve battery technology for our British artificial heart we were simply ignored.

Sure enough the knee jerk approach to sick patients was soon contributing to the UK's poor survival rates. The Covid-19 Hospitalisation in England Surveillance System actually showed the intensive care unit of admission to be a risk factor for death equally as strong as older age, pre-existing heart disease, and the presence of pre-existing immunosuppression. On Friday 4 September 2020, the *Daily Telegraph* wrote: 'Intensive care death rates dropped as doctors rejected ventilators.' Sure enough the 'ventilators and volunteers' strategy had cost lives, so what were the facts?

Before the first peak of infection rates on 1 April 2020, the Intensive Care National Audit and Research Centre showed that 76% of patients admitted to intensive care were soon intubated and ventilated. After the peak this number fell to 44% with the corresponding death rate dropping from 43% to 34%. In the interim, no new drugs were introduced nor were better clinical guidelines issued. The Department of Health suggested that the improvement followed 'informal learning.' The truth was that both China and Italy kept emphasising that high inflation pressures destroyed Covid-inflamed lungs. We had known that for forty years in cardiac surgery but still, sophisticated, less invasive breathing aids were not made available on the NHS. We even tried to persuade St Thomas' to use hydroxy gas for the Prime Minister, but to no avail. I suspect there was no money left. It had all been spent on useless ventilators which remained in warehouses and in Nightingale Hospitals that were never utilised. The reason was obvious. There were no staff to run them.

When things go badly in surgery, we employ a hypothetical instrument to shed light on what could have been done better. We call it the 'retrospectoscope'; while physicians refer to the process as reflection. In 2016, a simulated pandemic named 'Exercise Cygnus' showed that the NHS would be completely overwhelmed by a real life equivalent. The NHS Medical Director at the time commented upon a serious shortage of intensive care beds but the government considered the facts far too sensitive to be made public. Of course, silence was a sure route to the honours list. Don't rock the boat is the name of the game should you wish to represent the British Empire. Lessons learned during Cygnus were ignored and the public paid the price. Second hand shop health care.

The predictions were borne out by the catastrophic failures of the Covid effort. In England we had just 4,123 NHS intensive care beds which amounts to 6.6 per 100,000 population, and half the European average. Italy has 12.5 per 100,000 and Germany 29.2 per 100,000, virtually five times as many. Far more worrying was the corresponding lack of trained medical and nursing staff, and the vital equipment to support those beds. We didn't have either. The maximum surge capacity for ECMO in the whole country was thirty beds situated in five separate cardiac centres. That is a negligible number from an epidemiological standpoint, just something for the television to talk about as the body count escalated. I had retired so there was no longer any ECMO in Oxford where we pioneered it. As I argued in the medical press, why shouldn't every cardiac unit be equipped to save lives during their routine work? When the Prime Minister needed hospital admission in a deteriorating state, he was managed by the ECMO team at St Thomas'. Mercifully he didn't need it, but the vast majority who did were never given the chance.

Within weeks, the UK's Covid mortality rate stood at 182 patients per million versus Germany's 42 per million. Put another way, Germany had five times the critical care resources, including ECMO, and one fifth of the deaths. Once again, why is the NHS said to be the envy of the world when Taiwan, Hong Kong and Singapore performed much better on China's doorstep? Of course that was never discussed. What we got was propaganda. 'Clap for carers,' on the doorstep. When the virus reached the UK through our airports, there were 43,000 nursing vacancies and 100,000 NHS posts unfilled.

Covid killed 100,000 people through lung and multi-organ failure in 2020 alone. Of course, the doctors, nurses and technical staff we did have made heroic efforts under terribly difficult circumstances. When members of the Doctors Association were polled with the question 'do you feel that the NHS was prepared for Coronavirus?,' 99.5% of responders replied 'No.' That hardly inspired confidence, nor did the availability of personal protective equipment. A 'Dad's Army' of retired medical staff, including members of my own family, went back to the wards but it was difficult to make a difference without any acknowledged treatment for the lung failure. And of course, some of those doctors died.

Then in October came the headline 'Patients being brought back from the brink by reducing their immune system.' This was the news that certain drugs had specifically prevented the complement system from activating white blood cells thus protecting from the damage they caused. It was an 'I told you so' moment, forty years after my landmark article 'Complement and the damaging effects of cardiopulmonary bypass' from Alabama. This was six months and 50,000 deaths after I had tried to suggest the use of steroids from the standpoint of a well-meaning observer.

To quote those reinventing the wheel, 'switching off C5 can have a big effect. We and others have used anti-C5 blocking agents on very severe Covid patients with very promising results.' That is precisely what we achieved in heart surgery by identifying the harmful materials in the bypass circuit that triggered complement activation and having them replaced. It was C5 that I had measured for the first time in bypass patients. And just as we had employed steroids all those years ago, dexamethasone became the treatment of choice for Covid-19.

I presented my arguments again in a surgical journal. The title of the paper was 'A cardiac surgeon's perspective on the treatment of Coronavirus' with the subtitle 'Can interventions that surgeons use for prophylaxis protect against the cytokine storm?' Of course this had no influence. The pandemic was being managed by a committee of wise men whose eyes were closed to all but their own concepts. The small number of eminent virologists and statisticians provided their best advice to the government and sadly a huge pile of bodies followed.

Two years after my return from Wuhan, the UK had recorded 10,500,000 cases of Covid-19 with 150,000 deaths, equivalent to the city of Oxford. That exceeded 2000 deaths per million population, the highest mortality

TRAUMA OF A DIFFERENT KIND

in Europe and similar to Mexico, Chile, Latvia and the Ukraine. It was now double that of Germany, the Netherlands and Canada. Having promptly employed draconian measures, China recorded just 111,413 cases with three deaths per million population, though some considered those figures to be an underestimate. For Australia, New Zealand, Japan and Singapore the equivalent deaths per million were 79, 9, 145 and 127 respectively. Perhaps we should envy their health care systems and look closely at our own. Seriously.

So what had gone wrong? Foremost was the fact that the NHS was stretched to the limit long before the pandemic hit us and to disregard the findings of Exercise Cygnus left Britain extremely vulnerable. Then there was the inordinate delay in lockdown in the face of impending disaster. The worrying evidence from Wuhan and Italy was clear to see but still the borders were kept open.

Where was our capacity to test, trace and isolate cases as others had done? Initially there was abject confusion over the policies of lockdown versus herd immunity, then delay in acknowledging the full range of Covid symptoms. Deaths of untested victims in the community were left out of the statistics and, in desperation to liberate hospital beds, 25,000 elderly patients of undetermined Covid-19 status were transferred from hospitals to care homes. Carnage in the name of 'protecting the NHS.' The NHS needed protection because, as most of us knew, it was teetering on the edge of collapse before Covid arrived.

The Scripps Institute in California, who worked with me on the pivotal Alabama complement activation studies, analysed findings from a number of uniquely restricted environments including the Diamond Princess cruise liner, the USS Theodore Roosevelt and the whole population of Iceland. They showed that in 40% of cases the virus had been transmitted by fully asymptomatic carriers who would not feature in the British 'Test and Trace' system. Yet even those asymptomatic people showed evidence of lung damage on computerised tomography scans. So were our leaders following the appropriate science when they rammed it down our throats on BBC television every evening?

As Covid completely overwhelmed hospital services, some of us remained concerned for patients with heart disease and cancer. Compared with the eighteen months preceding the pandemic, the six months between July and December 2020 saw two million fewer hospital appointments and 27 million fewer visits to the general practitioner. As a result, 16,000 fewer cancer treatments were initiated while heart, brain and plastic surgery that relied upon critical care beds were forced to close.

The eminent cancer doctor, Professor Karol Sikora, along with the Queen's cardiologist, Professor Kim Fox, and I, published an article in the *Telegraph* newspaper entitled 'The NHS must remain open to all patients.' We wrote 'to close down the National Health Service will leave tens of thousands of patients with heart disease and cancer both frightened and hopelessly isolated. As a result, many will suffer and die prematurely. Their families will never forget this. Neither China nor Italy stopped treating serious conditions despite the chaos there earlier this year.'

There were good reasons for making this public statement. By December 2021, a damning report by the National Audit Office calculated that 740,000

TRAUMA OF A DIFFERENT KIND

cancer cases which should have been urgently referred by GPs had been missed since the first lockdown. And regrettably for cancer patients, a four week delay in treatment translates into a 10% fall in survival probability. Those who are not treated while potentially curable will usually die after four or five years when they could otherwise have lived.

Britain was languishing at the bottom of the cancer league tables even before Covid. Research by the World Health Organisation showed we had the lowest survival rates for five in seven common cancers. Indeed, some of our survival figures are worse than other European countries twenty years ago. We rank bottom of the table for bowel, lung, stomach, rectal and pancreatic cancer, second worst for oesophageal tumours and in third worst position for ovarian cancer. When early detection and tumour staging are the keys to survival, where do remote GP consultations and low numbers of computerised tomography and magnetic resonance imaging scanners leave us? British scientists were responsible for their development, but our use of the technology falls well below the European standards. On a par with Serbia and North Macedonia, in fact. 'Second hand shop' for the sake of being free at the point of delivery.

Patients with heart disease fared no better in the pandemic. Heart surgery virtually stopped apart from dire emergencies and was still bumping along the bottom two years later. Catheter laboratories closed with staff re-assigned to Covid roles, so coronary angioplasty and the use of catheter deployed heart valves were brought to a halt. By Autumn 2021, the British Heart Foundation calculated that more than 275,000 symptomatic cardiac

263

patients were left waiting for investigations and treatment. In the words of their Medical Director 'we saw growing waiting lists even before the pandemic. Now the pressure on the NHS has grown and the scale of the current cardiovascular crisis is unsustainable.' And that precedes the long term cardiac effects of Covid itself. So what did the government's slogan 'Protect the NHS' really mean? It spelled out 'sacrifice yourselves for a system that can't cope.' Tough unless you can afford private healthcare.

Covid decimated access to primary care, so much so that many of us now view GP surgeries as 'no go' areas. Universally there are long waits on the telephone to speak to a non-medical receptionist who will then make the judgement as to whether contact with a doctor is warranted. In desperation, many give up and take off for the nearest accident department. These are already inundated by the walking wounded who should be managed in general practice. Anxious souls and the elderly call an ambulance, wait endlessly and queue for hours outside the hospital before unloading. And while ambulances wait in line they are out of action for other patients who need them. As a result, the emergency treatment of heart attack and stroke patients in a catheter laboratory cannot happen. The damage is done and the public suffer for it.

Finally, let's return to the critically time dependent treatment of serious injuries, an issue I fought for throughout my career.

During 2021, all ten of England's NHS Ambulance Trust reported stress levels at their highest 'black alert.' Many repeatedly declared critical incidents resulting in the military being recruited to help them cope with

TRAUMA OF A DIFFERENT KIND

999 calls. Experienced paramedics reported marked personal distress when they lost patients simply through delay in unloading them. In other words the process of rescue for injured patients had disintegrated. Bye bye Golden Hour.

Between January and August 2021, the ambulance service reported 333 severe harm or death incidents, a 26% rise since the pandemic began, with most directly attributed to delays arriving at the scene or unloading in a reasonable time frame. In the month of July alone there were an extraordinary one million 999 calls and the system couldn't cope. Ambulance response times for the most pressing of circumstances such as cardiac arrest routinely exceed the eight-minute target. For the next category of urgency patients in London might wait four hours, and some regions faced delays of ten hours to deliver patients with a stroke or heart attack. This would amount to criminal negligence in anything but a state run system.

In October 2021, ambulances in the West Midlands were delayed outside hospitals for a cumulative total of 28,000 hours with an average of seventy-eight crews being unable to respond to 999 calls. Worse still, patients were dying in parked ambulances without having benefitted from emergency hospital treatment. The general public were asked to volunteer to convey 999 patients to the Emergency Department.

Let me explain how this impacted me from a personal perspective. Why I felt so strongly about it. I happened to be on the spot when a partially sighted pedestrian was hit by a motorcycle on a busy road in Oxfordshire. Fortunately, the rider had begun to decelerate towards a roundabout and came to an abrupt halt on impact

THE TRAUMA CHRONICLES

with the victim. I found her lying prostrate in the wet road against the front wheel. Now I was faced with a conscious woman in pain on the road, with rush hour traffic determined to pass the stationary obstruction. She did not appear to have fractured limbs so my judgement was that she would be safer moved to the pavement away from the flow of traffic.

I asked another bystander to assist me in carrying her while we supported the head and neck. Then I called 999 in the knowledge that there was a major ambulance depot just one mile away. The usual, tedious, time-consuming inquisition followed. The tick box stuff played out repeatedly on sensationalised television programmes where patient confidentiality is seemingly of no consequence. They have to do it but, at the other end of the line in a desperate situation, it is excruciatingly frustrating. In desperate straits all you want to see is the flashing blue lights rushing towards you. But no.

The police arrived quickly and were kind but the poor woman continued to lie uncomfortably on the cold pavement, shivering in distress and unable to communicate. We would learn that she had a fractured pelvis and was lapsing into shock. Soon I couldn't feel a pulse and she was gasping for air. That had been the ambulance controllers first question 'Is the patient breathing?' When I said 'yes' the word had immediately downgraded us in the pecking order. So we waited. And waited. And waited in the cold and dark.

It was more than an hour before the ambulance arrived, and of course the bystanders were hostile towards the crew for taking so long. The paramedics were apologetic but defensive, citing the unrelenting pressure on a system that couldn't cope. Should they put up a drip on site?

TRAUMA OF A DIFFERENT KIND

What good would that do? She was already hypothermic and further delay to push in cold clear fluid was irrational and would not help her. Why waste even more time when the accident department was only ten minutes away, so I urged them to move on. Reluctantly they agreed without my having to play the 'I am a doctor' card which I detest. A 'geriatric first aider' was a more apt description that evening and there were grumblings that I should never have moved her from the road in the first place.

As the blue lights disappeared towards Oxford, I felt infinitely sad. Sad for the woman and sad for the dismal state of a health service that I and other family members had served tirelessly for fifty years. It is a well-intentioned but broken model characterised by cost containment rather than 'clinical excellence' which the bureaucrats constantly allude to. It is simply not the way it used to be.

That grim episode by the roadside was the antithesis of what my colleagues at the Royal College of Surgeons had hoped for when we sought to improve trauma care. We were in Oxford, not the Outer Hebrides. The term 'Golden Hour' was coined decades ago for good reason yet we are now so resigned to mediocrity that nothing remarkable was seen in the delay. Nothing remarkable is seen in the cancellation of thousands of operations and cancer treatments nor the fact that those who can afford it are indeed flocking to the welcoming private sector. And remember, this alternative is predominantly staffed by NHS physicians and surgeons in their so called 'spare time.' Increasingly spare time as it seems.

We are left with sobering statistics. Currently an estimated nine million people are waiting for NHS treatment. The National Audit Office cautions that 'if 50% of missing hospital referrals return to the NHS and activity grows only in line with pre-pandemic levels, the waiting list will reach 12 million patients by 2025. Should 50% of missing referrals return and the NHS succeeds in increasing its activity by 10% more than planned, the waiting list will still be 7 million.'

Despite diversionary political banter, the UK simply does not have the doctors, nurses nor hospitals to cope with the workload. In 2018 we imported more doctors than we trained, many from third world countries that could ill afford to lose them. In 2019 this figure was an appalling 60%. At the peak of the pandemic in 2020, 30% of beds were occupied by Covid patients. Two years later, this proportion has fallen to 5%, but the system is still failing to cope. Woefully failing. One reason is that the number of inpatient beds has actually fallen drastically through the need to accommodate social distancing on the wards. So patients wait hours or days in the accident department for a bed while the ambulances queue to unload their emergencies—sometimes for eight hours or more, a whole shift time. In consequence, protracted ambulance response times decimate the crucially time dependent treatments to save victims of heart attack and stroke. Brain and heart muscle die minute upon minute.

'Is the patient breathing?' asks the call handler.

'Yes but they won't be by the time you get here,' comes the wry reply.

Of course this situation is not a subject for mirth. In an emotional debate in the House of Lords dire personal experiences were related by individual peers. Lord Robert Winston, an esteemed colleague from the Hammersmith

TRAUMA OF A DIFFERENT KIND

Hospital and one of Britain's most eminent medical scientists provided the saddest example. Lady Winston suffered a sudden cardiac arrest at home which caused him to make frantic attempts at resuscitation. Alone and in need of immediate help he paused the cardiac compressions to call an ambulance. He was then subject to the rote litany of irrelevant questions while he desperately attempted to dispatch more blood to the oxygen deprived brain. As Winston explained to the House 'the man asked me to count the number of heart beats per minute [but she had no cardiac contractions]. The waste of time is critical. When the man eventually backed down it was obvious that he had not been trained to ask the right questions!'

Raising the issue of ambulance handover delays the former BBC governor Lord Young related the case of another peer's son who had waited almost six hours to be taken to hospital after a stroke. His Lordship lamented, 'people are dying as we sit here in this chamber, literally thousands of them. Why? Because paramedics are waiting with trolleys in hospitals waiting for a bed. It's a national disgrace.'

How did the Health Minister, Lord Kamall, respond to the numerous complaints? 'Clearly there are too many incidents of this kind.' Followed by, 'We have an NHS action plan for urgent and emergency care which includes paramedics, the recruitment and retention of staff, and more space in Accident and Emergency Departments.' Sad. How often do we hear these excuses? We had great plans many years ago and look where we are now. Covid is not an excuse and money isn't the answer. We need a system that is accountable in a way that does not happen now.

THE TRAUMA CHRONICLES

Alluding to the widespread demise of patient care, on June 22, 2022 the *Daily Telegraph* reported on 'Scandal after scandal, waste after waste and death after death.' That same week the *British Medical Journal* piled in. 'We need a radical overall of safety. Individual hospitals or staff are blamed (for adverse events) - but the fish rots from the head!'

The perpetually spiralling clinical negligence bill is testament to this. It had reached £2.2 billion per year by 2020 before Covid struck but so fragile was the NHS that it soon shattered like a glass vase tumbling from the mantelpiece. Yet there is still no political will nor the guts to change it. The invariable retort is that 'we are putting in record levels of funding, appointing more managers, and writing vital reports on equality and diversity. Admirable but the fact is that 42% of medical staff are already from BAME backgrounds compared with 14% of the general population so who is deciding the priorities? Where do the suffering patients who lose their lives come into all this? This is not my criticism. It is the prevailing mood of the day. We signed up to save lives not lose them. It all used to be awfully simple in the old days. Now it's simply awful!' Simply awful when, with appropriate resources, it could be awfully simple.

The NHS began in 1948, the year that I was born. Sadly, neither of us remain fit for purpose and we urgently need repair. The politicians recognise that fact, yet no one dare move on it. Meanwhile, the sacred old cow continues to graze aimlessly and pass wind on those who care about it. Ironic that on New Year's Day, 2022, as our ground-breaking Covid mortality topped 150,000, those charged with managing the response

TRAUMA OF A DIFFERENT KIND

received their gongs. It was the same honours list attended by the architect of the Iraq war. The man who mistakenly spoke of weapons of mass destruction and triggered as many deaths as Covid did in Britain. As the old song says 'that's the way it is...'

271

POSTSCRIPT

It always seems impossible until it's done.

Nelson Mandela

Whether they were the good old days or times to be forgotten, the era of the fearless swashbuckling surgeon has passed. What's more, the contemporary profession openly celebrates that fact. So concerned were the Royal College of Surgeons about their macho image that the President, Neil Mortensen, a friend and colleague from Oxford, commissioned an enquiry about it.

Practically no one these days has sufficient training to intervene in more than one body cavity or in both adults and children. Most beneath consultant grade are now afraid to do anything independently. Contemporary training produces such micro specialists that in my own sphere there are dedicated mitral valve, aortic valve and coronary bypass surgeons. Deaths must be avoided at all costs since outcomes are published in the public arena. Of course, the direct route to negligible mortality is to avoid operating on the sickest patients. So why did a proud profession change so dramatically?

Thanks to the European Working Time Directive, those newly appointed as consultants have averaged just 6000 hours of hands-on surgical experience in an operating theatre. Moreover, the opportunities for a trainee to operate independently were decimated by a lethal name and shame policy dictated by NHS England long after the US had recognised the folly therein. If a consultant cardiac surgeon records a death, either by his own hand or through a trainee, it will be a long time before he is prepared to delegate another case.

Why did I lack inhibitions and self-doubt during my career? I guess it could have been attributed to the head injury, my 'Phineas Gage' moment. More likely it may have emerged through the confidence that builds through hands-on experience at the coal face. Before being taken on to develop cardiac surgery in Oxford, I'd personally accrued more than 40,000 hours of operating time during seven years as a senior registrar in London and the US. Any stress I may have suffered in the operating theatre was dissipated amidst that hard graft. There's a saying 'practice makes perfect' then another, 'nobody's perfect' and that included me. But I was experienced.

On the subject of 'stress and the surgeon', a retired colleague recently published a letter in the Bulletin of the Royal College of Surgeons which questioned the gentler 'touchy-feely' nature of training today. Provocatively, he opened his letter by asking 'are the right sort of people becoming surgeons and are they doing enough meaningful surgery to warrant the title of consultant surgeon?' The letter was written in response to an edition of the Bulletin dedicated to the raft of psychological support allegedly needed to keep surgeons afloat these days. Emphasising the gap between now and then his reminiscence reported that:

In my youth the consultant was god, and as such the hospital would acquiesce to their requests. Now that we have the "team" verses the "gallery" (meaning administrators) who feel it is their place to make

POSTSCRIPT

interventions, it makes it much more stressful for the surgeon to have to explain themselves every time they wish to do something a little out of the ordinary. Sometimes that really is a stress unless one is very well versed in one's subject and has a thick enough skin to do what you know to be the best.

Needless to say, that old fashioned stiff upper lip approach went down like a lead balloon and was panned mercilessly in reams of indignant responses in the next edition. One consortium of angry authors wrote 'what this letter so spectacularly fails to acknowledge is the real mental, physical and financial cost of burnout, anxiety and depression that evidence shows is prevalent amongst surgeons. Instead, the author tries to blame those mental health issues on the poorly selected surgeons themselves, on their lack of surgical experience and on their lack of received respect.' Eloquent!

They followed with 'In publishing this letter and giving it such prominence in the Bulletin, its editors and the College are tacitly promoting dinosaurian attitudes to work, surgery status and mental health that should have been consigned to extinction.'

So much for free speech then. The authors concluded that 'surgeons are not gods, nor should they aspire to be.' To be honest, most of us were far from god like, nor wanted to be. Many of us were a bit devilish in fact. But without doubt the patients wished their heart to be operated upon by confident respected figures — the introspective, results-orientated approach cannot be the best for our sickest patients.

Alongside this torrent of criticism were articles that truly reflect the prevailing climate. They included 'think before you cut,' followed by 'taking a baby to the trauma symposium,' then 'if we can't get to theatre, we can't learn to operate'. In 2022 came the news that most surgeons were suffering performance anxiety in relation to their work, frequently with an effect on their mental health. The study published in Annals of Surgery reported that 65% of those interviewed felt anxiety at times had a negative effect on their technical ability. And there were significant gender differences with women suffering the most. Being watched by other surgeons seemed to disturb many. Strange. I loved operating for audiences, auditoriums full of them and the more complex the case the better. Perhaps it was the disinhibition that stemmed from brain injury or the arousal performance relationship the psychologists talk about. But it wasn't bravado. It was such a great privilege to teach, sharing my knowledge and experience for the good of others.

So were things really so bad in the past? I think the maligned old soldier had a point. In the old days we were consumed by fighting for the patients, setting our own problems aside. Did the long hours take their toll? No. The experience gained was our badge of honour. It was the key to my self-confidence. Did the patients suffer because of it? No. Had we screwed up we knew we wouldn't progress in our chosen specialty. Was I stressed by the blood and gore or human misery that trauma surgery inflicted upon me? Not at all. Heart surgery on tiny babies was considerably more taxing and emotive.

In these times of stringent political correctness what am I looking for when I need help? Do I care if my surgeon is macho, feminine, homosexual or trans? Not at all. I want competence experience, judgement and resilience. What I don't want is someone who has spent

POSTSCRIPT

half of their career not operating for some reason. I'd be happy with a robot or ape if they could guarantee survival in difficult circumstances. Others may not see it that way. Good luck.

Was my surgical impulsivity and lack of inhibitions really a form of psychopathy as Dutton suggested? Perhaps, but another rational explanation came to me unexpectedly on my return trip from South America. I was flicking through an inflight magazine whilst reflecting on the case with a glass of Merlot. And there it was, an article discussing the positive side of the neurodevelopmental condition Attention Deficit Hyperactivity Disorder, or ADHD as it is commonly referred to. I stress the word positive because 40% of the prison population are said to suffer from ADHD.

I was never a straight A student. Far from it. These days I would never have been accepted in medical school. I even failed anatomy in my first term. Quite simply, I believe that my determination to succeed as a young man came from the well documented hyperfocus element of ADHD. This also accounts for the fact that I eventually managed to pass exams because I was so determined to operate on hearts. Why? Because as an impressionable young schoolboy I watched my grandfather die miserably from heart failure. That's why I went on to pioneer artificial hearts.

Restless excitement-seeking behaviour surely fitted the bill. What's more, my markedly disorganised life was entirely reliant on two strong women. In the hospital, all I wanted to do was operate so my practice was managed by Sue who continually compensated for my chaotic approach and sent me to the right airport. When she

277

THE TRAUMA CHRONICLES

needed time off for an operation, I stupidly accepted invitations to lecture in Japan and South Africa on the same day.

Outside the operating theatre I was a useless and difficult character. I drove cars much too fast, screwed up numerous relationships and was overly competitive on the sports field, justifying the label psychopath. My home life became entirely reliant on Sister Beautiful who, in the wake of some interesting affairs of her own, came to test the waters in Alabama and decided to stay with me. She could have done much better. Having said that it was probably a relief to Sarah that I wasn't at home very often. To this day I have never engaged with computers, paid a utility bill, used a cash machine or lifted a motor car bonnet. I couldn't be bothered to learn the simple steps required. And I am hopeless with deadlines, paying fines, and all aspects of paperwork unless it's writing books or scientific papers which I did prolifically. I could fix people and write about it but nothing else.

Why introduce my ADHD diagnosis at the end of an eventful career? I do it to encourage the many whose young lives have been blighted by the problem. Those who are always in trouble and may never have experienced the same unrelenting focus that I had. The ADHD brain usually doesn't conform unless treated. Personally, I didn't take medication at the stage I was diagnosed. It was far too late for me. I had already weathered the frequent criticism of my unconventional and determined approach. Perhaps I operated fast because I became bored easily. Or had a weak bladder. I suspect ADHD accounted for my impatience and refusal to accept mediocracy, professional acquiescence and the need to conform.

POSTSCRIPT

When I did need to calm down I jogged, or more recently staggered, around the magnificent Blenheim Estate with my dogs. Emerging through the Bladon gate near the church yard I would pause breathless on the bench next to Churchill's grave. In the dark days of World War II, Winston urged the country "never, never, never give in". I adopted that sentiment for my trauma patients and, although not always, it usually paid dividends.

A Note on the Author

Stephen Westaby rose from a poor family in the north of England to become one of the world's top heart surgeons. A rugby injury sustained while still at medical school transformed his personality into a flamboyant, driven, ambitious and almost manic determination to succeed in his chosen specialty, thoracic surgery. Decades later he was diagnosed with ADHD (Attention Deficit Hyperactivity Disorder).

This drive for perfection in his profession (in spite of or because of ADHD) took him to the world-renowned Harefield Hospital, the foremost heart surgery centre in Birmingham, Alabama, the newly-created cardiothoracic centre in Oxford, and then in 2019 in Wuhan he was the first Western doctor to learn about Covid before the virus was identified. Westaby recounts his time training and working with the giants and pioneers of cardiac surgery, including Christiaan Barnard, Denton Cooley, and John Kirklin to name but a few.

His career was perhaps best characterised by Winston Churchill's 'Never, never, never give in' and this book chronicles the triumphs and failures of his surgical life, the lives saved and extended, the innovations (such as artificial hearts) he developed, and his research discoveries.

Following on from his two earlier best-selling works, this volume is written with humour, insight, and a doctor's reverence for life and his patients. *The Trauma Chronicles* is an unmissable memoir of one of Britain's and the world's foremost surgeons.